Vulvar Reconstruction Following Female Genital Mutilation/Cutting (FGM/C) and other Acquired Deformities

Dan mon O'Dey

Vulvar Reconstruction Following Female Genital Mutilation/Cutting (FGM/C) and other Acquired Deformities

Springer

Dan mon O'Dey
Department of Plastic, Reconstructive
and Aesthetic Surgery Hand Surgery
Center of Reconstructive Surgery of Female Gender Characteristics
Luisenhospital Aachen
Aachen
Nordrhein-Westfalen
Germany

ISBN 978-3-030-02166-5 ISBN 978-3-030-02168-9 (eBook)
https://doi.org/10.1007/978-3-030-02168-9

Library of Congress Control Number: 2018961583

This Springer imprint is published by the registered company Springer Nature Switzerland AG
The registered company address is: Gewerbestrasse 11, 6330 Cham, Switzerland

Preface

The outer female genital is a unique and likewise important anatomic region clearly justifying more than just general reconstructive insights. This region has significance for many reasons. Besides its importance for sexuality, reproduction, culture, and art, it takes a key role in feminine identity influencing psychophysical balance of the individual.

In contrast, acquired deformities of that region caused by medical or nonmedical reasons can greatly disturb the before-mentioned balance. Such deformities, therefore, are usually life-changing conditions for those being affected, as in contrast influenced positively by reconstruction.

There are different reasons resulting in vulvar deformity, such as vulvar dermatosis like lichen sclerosus et atrophicus, vulvar pemphigus, vulvar malignomas like vulvar intraepithelial neoplasias (VIN), carcinomas, congenital anomalies, or deformities deriving from ritual vulvar mutilations/cuttings known as Female Genital Mutilation/Cutting (FGM/C). Regarding those different reasons responsible for the distortion of the outer female genital, the residual anatomic correlate is frequently comparable among each other. From an anatomic point of view, therefore, it does not make a great difference if the deformity derives from ablative surgery or ritual cutting. The technical requirements for the reconstruction of form and function remain the same.

FGM/C is a worldwide problem affecting millions and millions of girls and women. It is reported to occur in nearly all parts of the world due to migration, but it is most prevalent in Africa, Asia, and the Middle East. This practice refers to all procedures involving partial or total removal of anatomic units and/or subunits of the external female genital or other injuries to that region performed for nonmedical reasons. Women, then, suffer from serious physical and psychological problems. Many of them die resulting from bleeding or infection. Communities that perform FGM/C, however, know to report a variety of social, cultural, mystical, and even religious reasons to do it. Nevertheless, FGM/C seems not to be clearly fixed officially to religious textbooks. The practice, however, clearly violates diverse human rights including the birth-given right of health, safety, self-determination, and physical integrity. According to the World Health Organization (WHO), genital cutting affects millions and millions of women around the globe, and the number is still rising [1].

Plastic surgery, as the specialty of changing physical conditions, is able to cure bodily harm deriving from different causes. It offers therapeutic options that have life-changing potential and therefore show positive effects on psychophysical balance of the patients. Recreating normal and attractive anatomic conditions, however, is demanding and needs a passionate interest in the specialty, pioneering spirit, innovative strength, in-depth understanding of the specific anatomy, advanced technical abilities including microsurgical skills, and knowledge of specialized procedures. It is critical to meet these requirements when intending to perform "anatomic reconstruction."

This book describes specialized reconstructive techniques invented by the author all of which can effectively be used to anatomically rebuild the outer female genital following acquired deformities with a special focus on reconstruction after female genital mutilation/cutting (FGM/C). Following an introduction, giving an overview of the subject, the main chapters deal with general as well as specific material including detailed anatomic information. With the help of high-quality videos, photographs, and illustrations, the reader receives in-depth information on microsurgical reconstruction of the clitoral tip with the NMCS-procedure (neurotizing and molding of the clitoral stump), prepuce reconstruction with the OD-flap (omega-domed flap), and reconstruction of the vulva as an aesthetic unit using the aOAP-flap (anterior obturator artery perforator flap) technique. The book is completed with chapters dealing with the problem management and postoperative care after complex vulvar reconstruction.

Moreover, based on many years of experience in medically dealing with FGM/C, this book is a personal view and statement on FGM/C.

Aachen, Germany Dan mon O'Dey

Reference

1. World Health Organization. Eliminating female genital mutilation: an interagency statement. Geneva: World Health Organization, Department of Reproductive Health and Research; 2008. p. 1–48.

Contents

Introduction

1

1.1 A General View

All over the world people share different traditions and rites. The resulting behavior is almost always believed to lead into improved fertility, health, or physical comfort. Some of the behaviors are also believed to be part of religious ideologies and/or spiritual practice, even though they may not be fixed officially to religious textbooks but carried further by varying reliabilities of oral or written traditions. Even the supposed relation to religion, however, may sometimes be counterproductive in terms of humanitarian rights and moral progress. Concerning different religions there might be people who care for tradition and those who care for religion. So religion and tradition might sometimes be separated from each other, and likewise influence each other, but not depend on each other. Fortunately it should be easier to alter tradition than religion.

Worldwide an incredible number of females are made to suffer from sexual offense and discrimination. These norms are usually anchored in the respective patriarchal culture and aim to control women's sexuality. Female genital mutilation/cutting (FGM/C), unfortunately, is such a practice being deeply rooted in traditional behavior. From a medical and/or humanitarian point of view FGM/C, therefore, is one of the biggest harms against women existing in the world today and likewise one of the most problematic culturally fixed burden that needs to be ended.

1.2 Female Genital Mutilation/Cutting (FGM/C)

FGM/C is performed entirely for nontherapeutic purposes. It comprises all procedures that cause partial or complete damage to different anatomic units and subunits of the outer female genital resulting primarily in graduated loss of form and

D. m. O´Dey, *Vulvar Reconstruction Following Female Genital Mutilation/ Cutting (FGM/C) and other Acquired Deformities*,
https://doi.org/10.1007/978-3-030-02168-9_1

function. Furthermore, chronic pain, inability of clitoral sensation, urinary disorders, fistulas, cysts, and recurrent infections are secondary effects impairing women's health.

Concerning my personal experiences with FGM/C I learned from the affected and people involved that it is more than only a ritual practice; it is a social attitude that subordinates women to men. The latter lastly results in sexual assault and oppression. This is one of the most long-lasting human errors.

The most common classification of FGM/C belongs to the World Health Organization (WHO) and was established in 2007. It comprises four basic types, which in turn are divided into different subtypes to cover a broad range of practices [1]:

Type I: Partial or total removal of the clitoris and/or clitoral prepuce ("clitoridectomy")
  Type Ia: Removal of the clitoral prepuce (Fig. 1.1a, b)
  Type Ib: Removal of the clitoris and the clitoral prepuce (Fig. 1.2)
Type II: Partial or total removal of the clitoris and the labia minora, with or without excision of the labia majora ("excision")

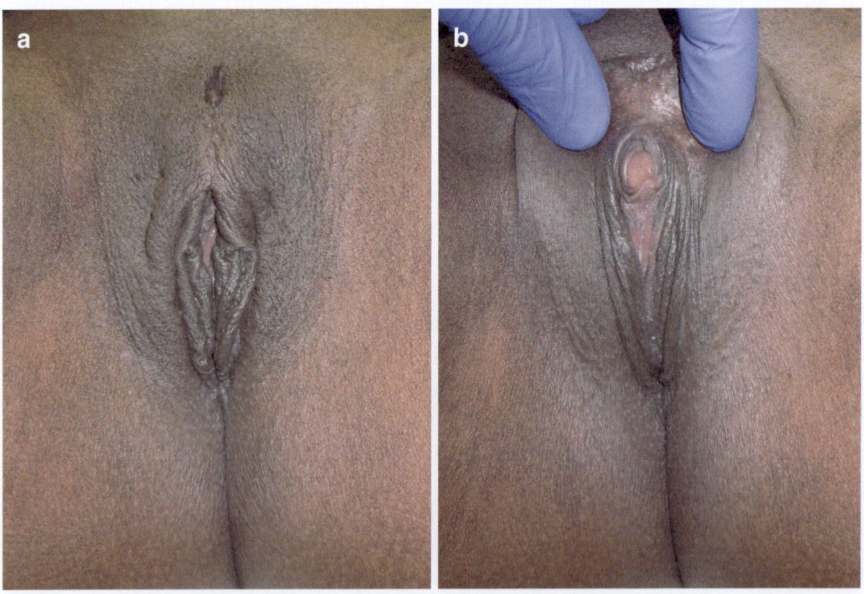

Fig. 1.1 35-Year-old woman showing a FGM/C type I (Ia) genital cutting with amputated and tightly adapted clitoral prepuce. (**a**) (left) Tissue at rest. (**b**) (right) Exposition of the covered clitoral tip through lifting up the scar in the region of the prepuce

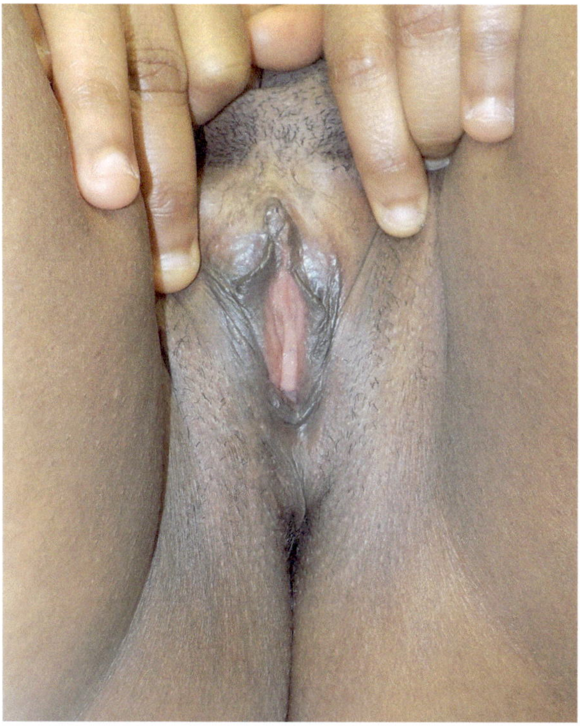

Fig. 1.2 23-Year-old woman showing a FGM/C type I (Ib) genital cutting with amputated clitoral tip and prepuce

Type IIa: Removal of the labia minora (Fig. 1.3)
Type IIb: Partial or total removal of the clitoris and the labia minora (Fig. 1.4)
Type IIc: Partial or total removal of the clitoris, the labia minora, and the labia majora (Fig. 1.5)

Type III: Narrowing of the vaginal orifice with creation of a covering seal by cutting and apposition of the labia minora and/or the labia majora, with or without excision of the clitoris ("infibulation")
Type IIIa: Removal and apposition of the labia minora (Fig. 1.6)
Type IIIb: Removal and apposition of the labia majora (Fig. 1.7)

Type IV: Unclassified: All other harmful procedures to the female genital for non-medical purposes, for example, pricking, piercing, incising, tearing, scraping, and cauterizing

Anatomically the term "total removal of the clitoris" used by the WHO does not mean removal of the whole organ comprising the glans (tip), the corpora (body), the crura, and the bulbs [see 2], but removal of the clitoral glans and part of the clitoral corpora. Fortunately, partial removal of the organ is the anatomic prerequisite warranting for functional reconstruction of the clitoral glans. This is even true for very

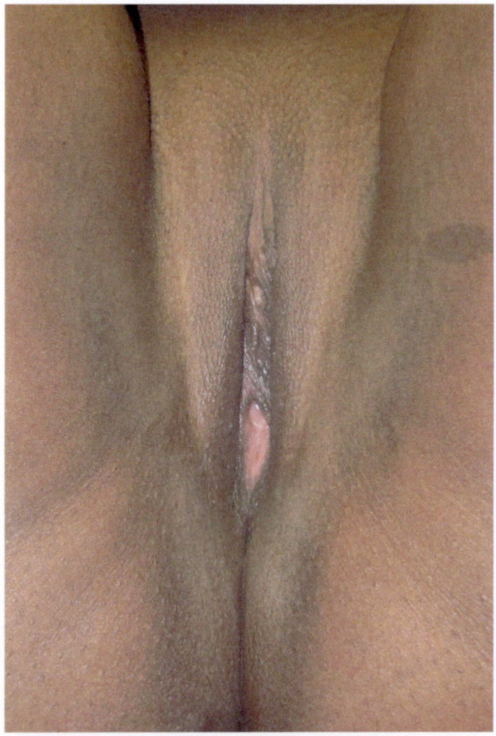

Fig. 1.3 27-Year-old woman showing a FGM/C type II (IIa) genital cutting with amputated and adapted minor labias; the clitoral tip is partly visible

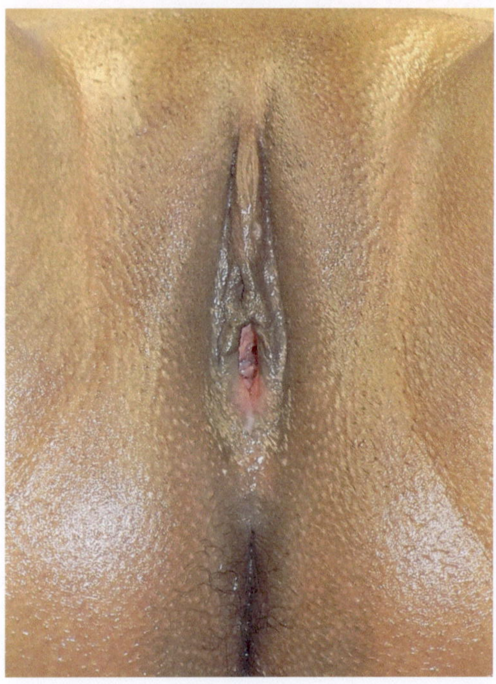

Fig. 1.4 20-Year-old woman showing a FGM/C type II (IIb) genital cutting with amputated and adapted minor labias, as well as amputated clitoral tip and prepuce

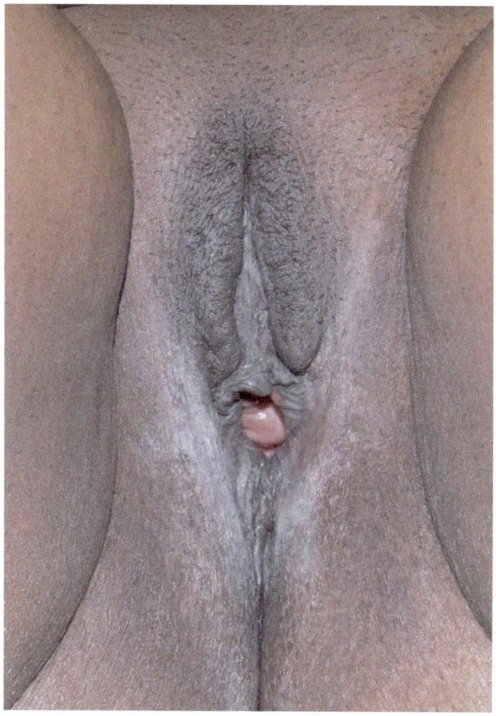

Fig. 1.5 40-Year-old woman showing a FGM/C type II (IIc) genital cutting with amputated clitoral tip and body, prepuce, minor and partly major labias in the adapted posterior part

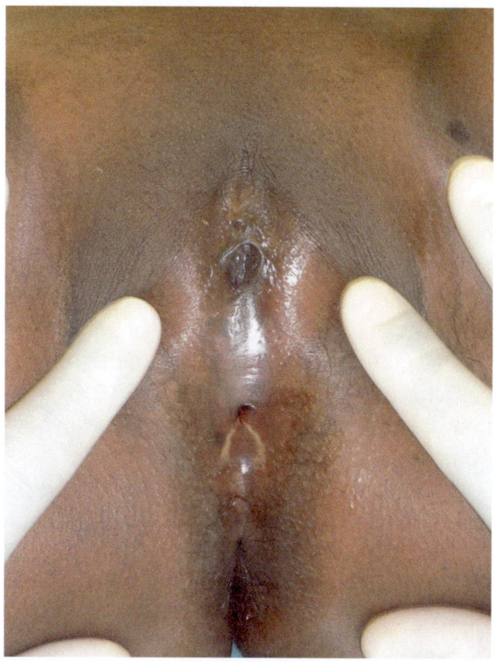

Fig. 1.6 37-Year-old woman showing a FGM/C type III (IIIa) genital cutting with amputated prepuce, clitoral tip, and minor labias, which are adapted to a minimal vaginal opening

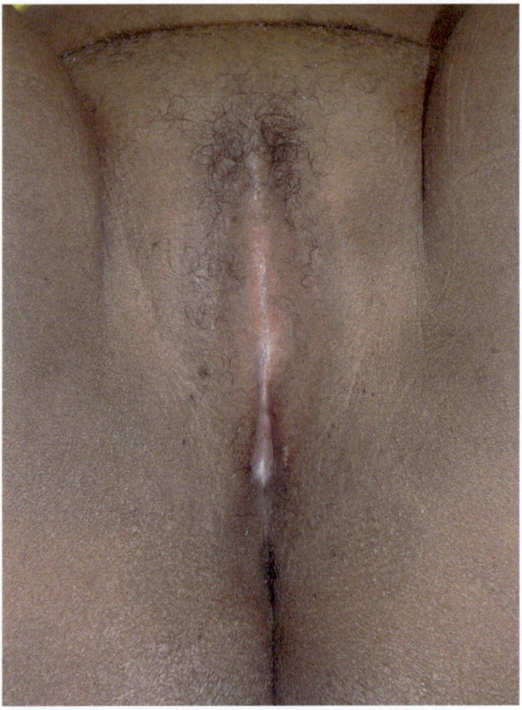

Fig. 1.7 36-Year-old woman showing a FGM/C type III (IIIb) genital cutting (infibulation) with amputated prepuce, clitoral tip, and minor and major labias that are adapted to a minimal vaginal opening

radical excisions performed all the way down to the pubic bone leaving behind only the clitoral crura. However, functional reconstruction of the clitoral tip then is also possible but marginal.

It is estimated that more than four million girls and women are genitally mutilated each year for nonmedical but only ritual reasons. Out of these rites, infibulation is worst and affects about 400,000 girls and women each year. The number of all affected females is that high that it can hardly be realized by one's mind. Relying on different publications there are more than 200,000,000 [3] girls and women affected by FGM/C around the world. Out of these it is estimated that a minimum of 500,000 girls and women are living in Europe and round about 180,000 are at risk [4]. Africa is mainly concerned, but also Asia and even Europe due to migration. Genital cutting is often done due to existing myths and tradition. Religion seems to be frequently associated with FGM/C, even though no official textbook does mention it. It is remarkable that FGM/C is anyhow widely regarded as a basic element of the respective religion.

FGM/C, however, is violence against girls and women; it is child abuse; it is a bodily mutilation; it is a significant psychological and physical injury, and it is clearly a kind of sexual offense. FGM/C subordinates females and oppresses their capacities and everyday behavior. FGM/C therefore is a kind of imposed captivity.

There are different effects believed being caused by FGM/C. It is thought, for example, that FGM/C reduces the sexual drive of women, likewise ensuring their virginity until marriage and loyalty to their forthcoming husband. It is also believed that it makes genitals cleaner, good looking, and socially more acceptable. For many reasons mothers often want their daughters to look the same as they do. In the Maasai tribe, for example, it is believed that an uncut clitoral region will lead into a poor harvest or an overall misfortune for the family and/or even the community. These existential concerns are of course relevant for the parents' decision to hand over their daughter for genital cutting even though they know that it will be very harmful for them. It is assumed that there is a significant mortality rate after infibulation due to bleeding, infection, or both. It is remarkable, however, that in case of a serious complication or a consecutive death following the procedure nobody tends to speak about it neither in the concerned community nor to the outside world. To this concern information is limited.

It is, however, thanks to education guided by public institutions in cooperation with diverse groups and initiatives of civil and medical society, that some communities change their traditional attitude and do abandon the practice. Traditional change, though, is often a very slow process. Regarding the Maasai tribe the most important and leveraging effect to eliminate FGM/C is to convince influential community members such as community elders or other respected people. All members of the community will usually follow the attitude of these leading people without any concerns. In many countries FGM/C is performed though the law prohibits it. In those communities no one will call the procedure into question and will also never tell about it outside of the community. So, the law only does not abandon FGM and does obviously not relieve people from it. The main focus therefore remains on education by convincing people that it is a harmful and useless procedure, and that myths have nothing to do with reality.

Economy plays also an important role. Parents worry that their uncut daughter might not be accepted by the community, be socially excluded, be considered as unmarriageable, and therefore are financially unsecured. A shift of values or kind of economic alternatives must be created for those families refusing genital cutting especially in communities where grants are existentially for the bride's family (Fig. 1.8). This will bring further motivation to abandon genital cutting. School education and professional training are important values creating economic independency. But all these efforts will not have a lasting effect if they cannot effectively be implemented into the community's tradition. That is why progress evolves unfortunately slow.

There is a debate if the practice of female genital cutting should generally be regarded as mutilation or if less severe forms, such as rubbing genitals with herbs or pricks, might be tolerated especially when physicians perform it. Well, every form of genital cutting, if neither medically indicated, nor of the personal intention, is harm. FGM/C is therefore unethical. It is a non-willing procedure and does clearly result in physical and psychological injury. Moreover, it is physical and psychological violence and should never ever be regarded as culturally given. In contrast, it

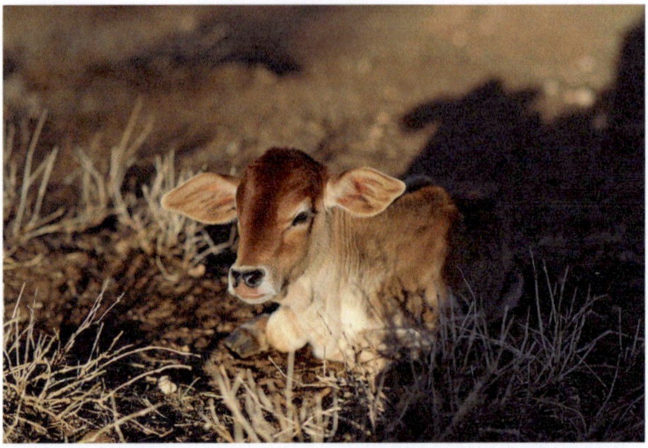

Fig. 1.8 "The gift." A Tanzanian calf serving as a typical dowry in the Maasai tribe

must be definitively antagonized. Neither medicalization nor toleration of FGM/C is an option but eradication. Female genital mutilation/cutting has no benefits, causes only harm, and might be regarded as one of the most problematic attitudes of which females are made to suffer today.

1.3 Personal Trip to Tanzania

When I traveled to Tanzania in 2013, joining a group of courageous women active in the fight against FGM/C, the intention was to get an idea about cultural backgrounds of FGM/C, and medical care following complications. On-site we joined activists of NAFGEM (Network Against Female Genital Mutilation) and visited different villages of the Maasai tribe, women's refuges, schools, physicians, and the biggest medical facility in Moshi. It was an incredibly intensive journey with lots of impressions and important insights. We met and talked to elders, parents, youth, families including husbands, brothers, sisters, uncles, aunts, grandmas, grandfathers, as well as circumcisers, teachers, doctors, activists against FGM/C, and of course affected girls and women. It was an amazing and likewise an important experience. Very soon it became obvious that FGM/C is deeply rooted and interwoven in a complex network of cultural, social, sexual, economic, and also religious backgrounds and last but not least firmly linked to tradition (Fig. 1.9).

Tradition itself reflects beliefs, values, and attitudes that can only be changed by conviction. Change, therefore, is very hard to establish in this context. Unfortunately, it is believed for example that FGM/C prepares girls for adulthood and/or marriage, protect them for losing their virginity un- or willingly, ensure their loyalty to their future husbands, make them bodily "clean," maintain the family's honor, as well as ensure social integrity and economic security.

Parent's belief to protect their daughters and to prepare them best possible for their future life by handing them over to the procedure of FGM/C. FGM/C, therefore, is a dilemma.

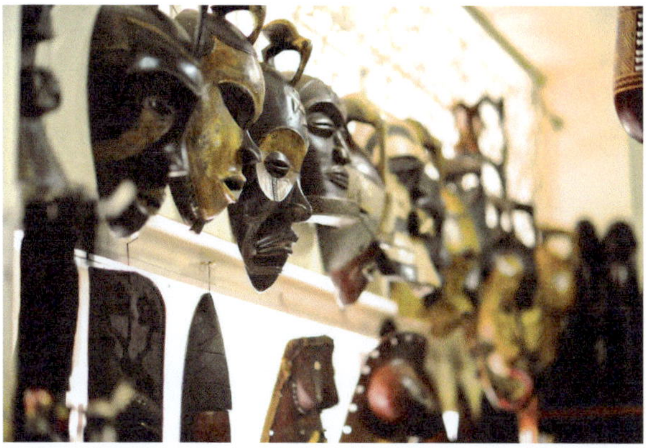

Fig. 1.9 "Masks." Typical Tanzanian masks reflecting mysteries and myths

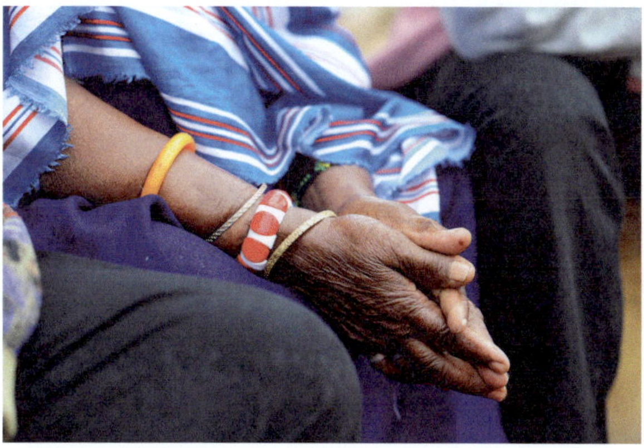

Fig. 1.10 "Hands." The hands of an old and retired Maasaian circumciser

In the Maasai tribe circumcisers are frequently older women who keep up with the tradition, and are additionally entrusted with other important duties like being midwives, and healers. Surprisingly, one very old woman (Fig. 1.10) that I got to know working as a circumciser though suffering from blindness and age states that she would never ever attend nor do any circumcisions again because she cannot stand screaming of the traumatized children any more (Fig. 1.11). Her point of view once more reflects that also circumcisers cannot be uncritically regarded as vicious or inhuman, but as people being both captured and driven by something called "*Tradition*."

In general it is not right to intend control of girl's and women's sexual and reproductive capacity by any means. So, a "*Tradition like FGM/C*" is not covered by immunity. It clearly offers room for a change. Tradition sometimes must be changed.

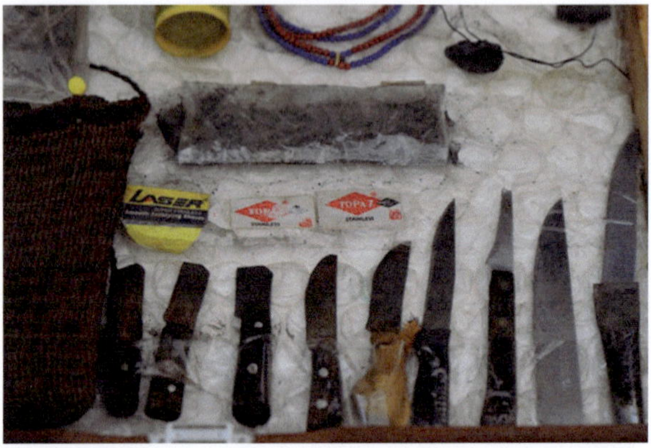

Fig. 1.11 "Knifes." Collection from NAFGEM (Network Against Female Genital Mutilation) of secured circumciser utilities from Tanzanian villages

1.4 The European Community and FGM/C

Concerning Europe, FGM/C is increasingly present due to the rising number of affected immigrants arriving from countries where FGM/C is commonly performed. In addition, it is believed that also unaffected girls living in Europe are taken back to their families' country of origin just for holidays to expose them to the rite of genital cutting. It shall be assumed that even sometimes circumcisers are flied into Europe for the procedure. Due to these diverse possibilities to be cut, protecting every girl and woman from the procedure is not easily done and likewise actually not possible regarding the current situation.

Dignity is a natural right of every human being and should be regarded as inviolable. It should be respected and saved by all human beings, especially by adults taking responsibility for younger people. Why should children, that do not even have an idea about sexuality, be bodily and mentally harmed by adults for sexual purposes and without any consent? This is fundamentally wrong and clearly violates dignity and self-determination of the affected.

1.5 The Ritual of FGM/C and Its Side Effects

Due to the raw experience most of the affected are exposed to, FGM/C shows some significant side effects on them, all of which may be physical or psychological in origin.

1.5.1 Physical and Psychological Damage

Concerning FGM/C, usually female adults forcibly hold children while the mutilation/cutting is performed with diverse cutting devices (Fig. 1.11). Beforehand children are usually made to believe that the procedure is a kind of celebration they can look forward to. Typically anesthetics are not used and that's why defense mechanisms of the children frequently lead into aggravation of the genital trauma. The legs are then usually bound together to promote healing of the cut edges and the children are forced to lie down for several days or weeks.

There are, of course, immediate and long-term complications resulting from the procedure that are serious to and frequently life changing for the affected girls and women. Victims usually feel deeply stigmatized even though physical damage caused by the procedure is usually not visible due to clothing. The simple awareness of being mutilated/cut does already cause enormous stress to the affected. That's why an unsuccessful procedure will also show long-term harm on the affected (see Sect. 1.5.2).

In children basic trust may be fundamentally disturbed and there can be many psychological consequences affecting mental balance including fear of sexual contact, stress disorders, anxiety, and depression. Further immediate complications comprise pain, shock, bleeding, wound infections, infections resulting from shared and unsterilized instruments, and death. Long-term complications include chronic pain resulting from neuromas and scars, recurrent infections resulting from epithelial inclusion cysts [5], abscesses, instable scars, urinary tract infections, discomfort resulting from sexual dysfunction, vulvovaginal trauma resulting from sexual intercourse and/or delivery, need for surgery to enable sexual intercourse ("defibulation"), delivery, vaginal and urinary outflow, or gynecological procedures requiring vaginal access.

FGM/C patients that I have seen in my office able to have sexual intercourse usually complain of sexual dysfunction due to tissue loss, reduced elasticity aggravated by scarring, cysts, and neuromas of the clitoral organ. Concerning the literature, however, "psychosexual dysfunction" in FGM/C patients seems to be debatable [6, 7]. Some confirm [6] and some deny [7] that most women suffering from FGM/C show sexual dysfunctions. The debate might be justified on both sides due to the fact that the clitoral organ is in general partly intact; there are multiple variants within the respective design of a FGM/C type I, type II, or type III procedure depending on the land or tribe of origin, and the sample sizes are usually imbalanced and/or small [7].

All in all, FGM/C is and remains a degrading, disabling, and disrespectful procedure to human beings that hopefully can be abandoned one time once and for all.

1.5.2 Psychological Damage Without Physical Correlate

Sometimes the mutilating/cutting procedure does not succeed due to many reasons including defense mechanisms of the affected, protective behavior of relatives, or fake practice by the circumcisers. Concerning my clinical experience, I occasionally see victims of FGM/C who do not show physical damage caused by the procedure, but do really belief that they were cut. These patients might remember that the FGM/C procedure was forcibly intended in their early childhood or that they might be deeply traumatized by just having attended the procedure. Remarks on their physical complaints are understandably mostly somewhat unclear, but they usually report on an unfulfilled sexual life and moreover show significant psychological burden. Of course reconstructive surgery is no answer for those patients, but particularly psychological support.

1.6 Other Acquired Deformities

Acquired vulvar deformities frequently result from ablative surgery. There are different pathologic changes in the squamous skin of the outer female genital or pathologies of adjacent structures of the vulva such as inflammation of the Bartholin glands that require medically indicated tissue removal leading to similar or even aggravated defects as those resulting from FGM/C. Changes of the skin include exemplarily nonneoplastic diseases, neoplastic diseases, inflammatory diseases, traumas, burns, scarring, soft-tissue contractures, and even non-rationable alterations like vulvodynia. Reconstructive needs following ablative surgery therefore are frequently comparable with those necessary for FGM/C patients and are oriented on the respective deformity. From an anatomic point of view the main problem resulting from ablative surgery is significant tissue loss showing complex reconstructive needs. The anticipated defect, the possible reconstructive options, and the expected reconstructive result considering form and function should be carefully reflected beforehand and also explained to the patient. Besides reconstruction, an interdisciplinary approach is sometimes required primarily or secondarily.

Due to defect similarity some important acquired deformities other than those resulting from FGM/C are described in the following.

1.6.1 Nonneoplastic Disorders

Pathologic skin alterations may necessitate partial or total resection of the vulva. Reconstruction of the vulva can be surgically best performed at the time of resection due to elasticity of the remaining tissue.

Lichen sclerosus et atrophicus is a frequent, inflammatory, and noninfectious dermatosis that in the long run might change into squamous cell carcinoma [8, 9]. However, till date there is no knowledge about the etiology of lichen, but it is assumed that it is based on an autoimmune disorder. It is one of those diseases which need further pioneer work concerning both basic research and therapeutic options [9]. The clinical problem with lichen sclerosis et atrophicus is complex. It leads into loss of the normal anatomy of the inner and outer vulva by fading and merging of its anatomic units and subunits. The minor and the inner part of the major labias may disappear in the long run, opening of the prepuce and thereby passing of the clitoral tip do coalesce (phimosis), and last but not least the vaginal entrance consecutively narrows accompanied by fissuring of the vulvar epithelium especially at the posterior commissure. The remaining vaginal opening is comparable with the condition following FGM/C type III. Tissue quality, however, is worse because of pathologic shrinkage, fibrosis, and consecutive loss of elasticity.

Apart from so-called porcelain white changes of the vulvar skin, sensory loss of the clitoral tip, and functional loss of the vaginal introitus, patients suffer from several complaints such as vulvar pruritus, burning sensations, recurrent fissuring of the vulvar skin resulting from mechanic irritations, or even spontaneous and disabling dyspareunia. Lichen sclerosus et atrophicus, therefore, has a lasting and impairing effect on the quality of life. It usually, however, does not affect other tissues apart from the vulva as it is observed in lichen ruber planus disease. The latter also affects other regions such as the vagina, other mucosas, and squamous epithelias.

Conservative treatment of lichen sclerosus et atrophicus is usually symptomatic and especially accomplished with local applications of highly potent corticosteroids; besides estrogens, and moisturizing substances. Especially long-lasting therapies with local corticosteroids can produce unintended secondary effects to the skin, like atrophy and vulnerability, leading to a vicious circle. Nevertheless, conservative treatment effects noticeable relief of symptoms from episode to episode. Healing, however, usually does not occur [10].

Operative treatment includes surgical separation followed by application of corticosteroid [11], local excision, or more extensive procedures like vulvectomy [8] followed by direct closure, mucosal advancement flaps, vulvar skin advancement, and mucosal or non-mucosal skin grafts [9]. Regarding anatomic reconstruction results are different. Grafts frequently tend to shrink and show loss of elasticity. Maintenance therapy with topical corticosteroids is recommended to prevent scarring, recurrence, and malignant alteration [12].

Concerning my clinical experience with the surgical treatment of lichen sclerosus et atrophicus in supposed advanced cases, complete excision accomplished by skinning vulvectomy and surface reconstruction with all-layered non-vulvar fasciocutaneous tissue, especially with the aOAP flap, is key to cure the disease, to control local recurrence, and to provide normal anatomic conditions for the patient. In case of lichen sclerosus et atrophicus it seems that "steel can heal." The challenge, however, remains then achieving normal anatomic conditions through the reconstructive procedure. With the aOAP flap technique normalized anatomic conditions can be achieved especially in extensive vulvectomy cases (Fig. 1.12a–f). Long-term personal follow-up reevaluations of more than 10 years show neither clinical recurrence of the disease nor return of any symptoms associated with it. Moreover, aOAP-flap vulvar reconstruction is able to normalize vulvar anatomy with regard to vaginal delivery. The latter is a very important perspective for patients in the fertile age.

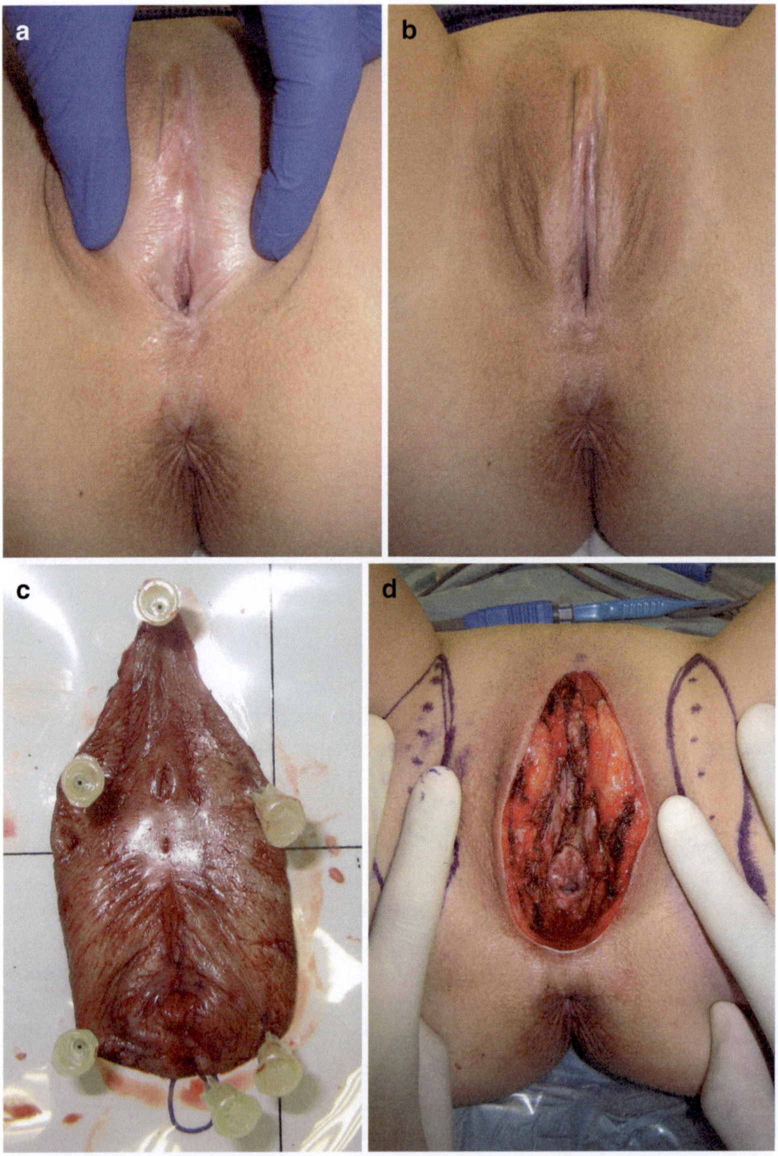

Fig. 1.12 28-Year-old woman with a late lichen sclerosus et atrophicus showing faded minor labias coalesced with the major labias, covered clitoral tip, and narrowed vaginal introitus. (**a**) (top left) Preoperative view of the outer genital. (**b**) (top right) Preoperative view of the outer genital with the major labias tightened up; note the faded clitoral region, minor labias, and narrowed vaginal introitus. (**c**) (middle left) Intraoperative view after partial vulvectomy of the diseased tissue. (**d**) (middle right) Intraoperative view following resection presenting with an extensive vulvar defect and marking of the both sided aOAP flaps on the genitofemoral sulcus. (**e**) (bottom left) 1-Year follow-up examination after aOAP vulvar reconstruction; note the natural aspect of the vulvar and inconspicuous scarring of both the harvest side and the vulva; form and function have turned to normal without recurrence of the disease. (**f**) (bottom right) 1-Year follow-up examination after aOAP-flap vulvar reconstruction showing the vulva in the upright position; note the normal contour of the vulva and inconspicuous scarring of the harvest side

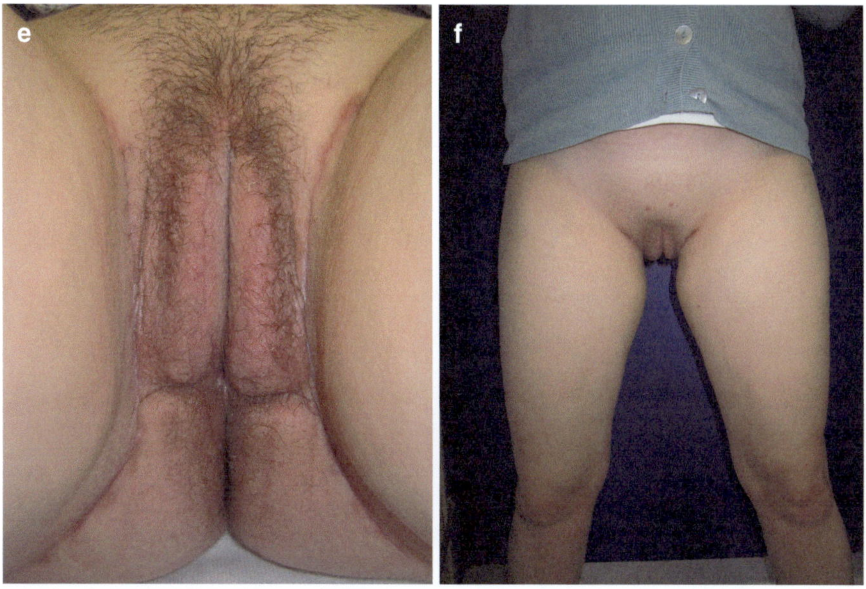

Fig. 12 (continued)

1.6.2 Neoplastic Disorders

Ablative surgery of vulvar neoplasias often leaves extensive defects that are difficult to reconstruct [13].

Neoplastic disorders include intraepithelial neoplasias also known as VIN I–III (vulvar intraepithelial neoplasias) lesions. The International Society of Vulvovaginal Disease (ISSVD) classified the severity of intraepithelial neoplasias according to the biology of the underlying neoplastic changes. As a result the known precancerous condition called VIN I skin lesion was ranked as a reactive and self-limiting epithelial irritation. VIN II and VIN III were changed into "usual type" and "differentiated type." The usual type especially includes diseases associated with HPV-16 (human papilloma virus) infections. The differentiated type comprises those lesions that were either not associated with HPV or associated with lichen sclerosus et atrophicus [14].

Nevertheless resection leaves complex defects and reconstruction is demanding. If the harvest side by means of the genitofemoral sulcus is not impaired by resection, aOAP-flap reconstruction is an effective option to reestablish form and function of the outer female genital in cancer patients (Figs. 1.13, 1.14, and 1.15). Especially in younger patients but also in older patients with sexual activity reestablishing normal sexual function and body image is crucial for life balance.

Reconstruction following resection can be performed at the same time or delayed depending on both the oncologic needs and the therapy concept. Adjuvant therapy like chemotherapy or radiation also impairs non-tumor healthy tissue important for reconstruction.

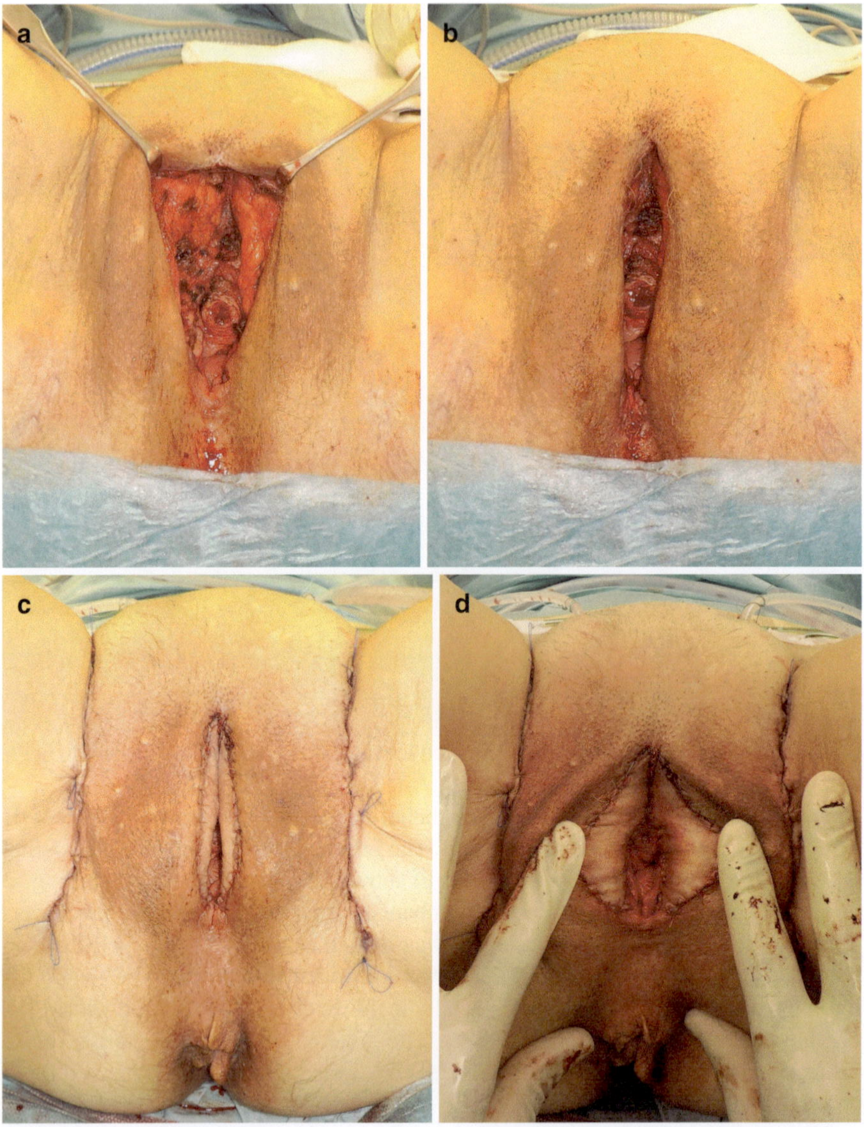

Fig. 1.13 76-Year-old woman with an extensive vulvar cancer of vulvar vestibule including region of the clitoral tip. (**a**) (top left) Intraoperative view after tumor excision including the region of the clitoral tip and the clitoral body showing extension of the defect. (**b**) (top right) Intraoperative view after partial vulvectomy showing the defect at rest. (**c**) (middle left) Intraoperative view after medially tunneled transposition of the both sided aOAP flaps and closure of the harvest side by means of a medial thigh lift. (**d**) (middle right) Intraoperative view after complete aOAP-flap inset demonstrating flexibility of the reconstructed vaginal introitus. (**e**) (bottom left) 1-Year follow-up examination after aOAP-flap vulvar reconstruction; note the natural aspect of the vulva and inconspicuous scarring of both the harvest side and the vulva; form and function have turned to normal without recurrence of the disease. (**f**) (bottom right) 1-Year follow-up examination after aOAP-flap vulvar reconstruction showing conditions in the upright position; note the normal contour of the vulva and inconspicuous scarring of the harvest side

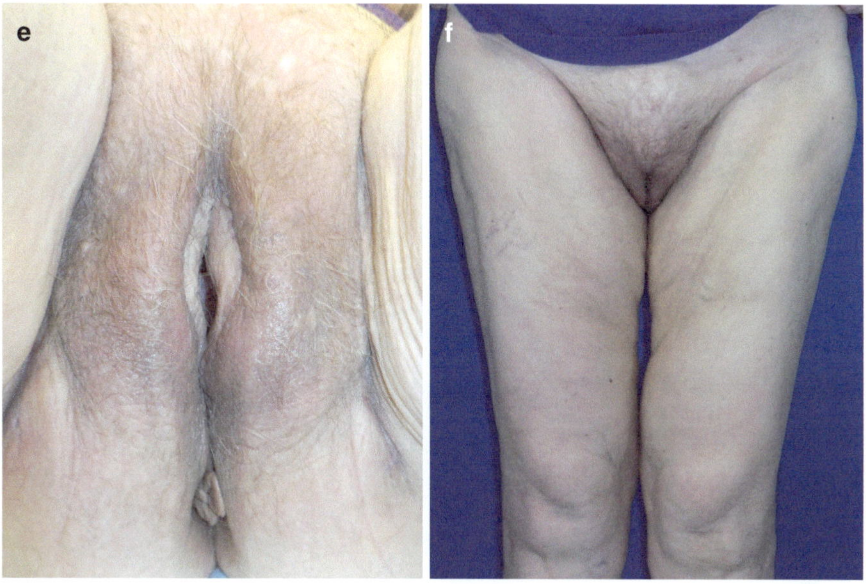

Fig. 13 (continued)

That's why immediate reconstruction often provides better tissue qualities concerning both the harvest and the recipient sides frequently showing better results. In addition scarring and the resulting contracture of soft tissue make the reconstruction more complex and somewhat less effective.

1.6.3 Inflammatory Diseases

Usually intact skin is a perfect barrier preventing microbiological invasion. Finest injuries to the skin, however, allow microbes to get through this barrier. Some of them are highly virulent and can cause serious systemic infections such as necrotizing fasciitis. Due to the loose subcutaneous tissue of the vulva, facilitating progressive microbial invasion, all inflammation even if superficial or abscesses should be considered as potentially serious. Any fluid from an abscess, of course, should be taken to a microbiological institute for Gram staining and processing for the identification of facultative and obligated anaerobic bacteria. For empiric treatment of vulvar infection the use of metronidazole and cefuroxime or clindamycin can be recommended [15].

Vulvar folliculitis, showing resistance to conservative therapies, can lead to partial or full vulvectomy making reconstructive surgery finally necessary. Procedures used for reconstruction depend on the involvement of surrounding tissue. If the genitofemoral sulcus is free of inflammation, it is one of the best options available for vulvar reconstruction. Depilation of the flaps before or after the procedure may be crucial for stable and recurrence-free long-lasting results.

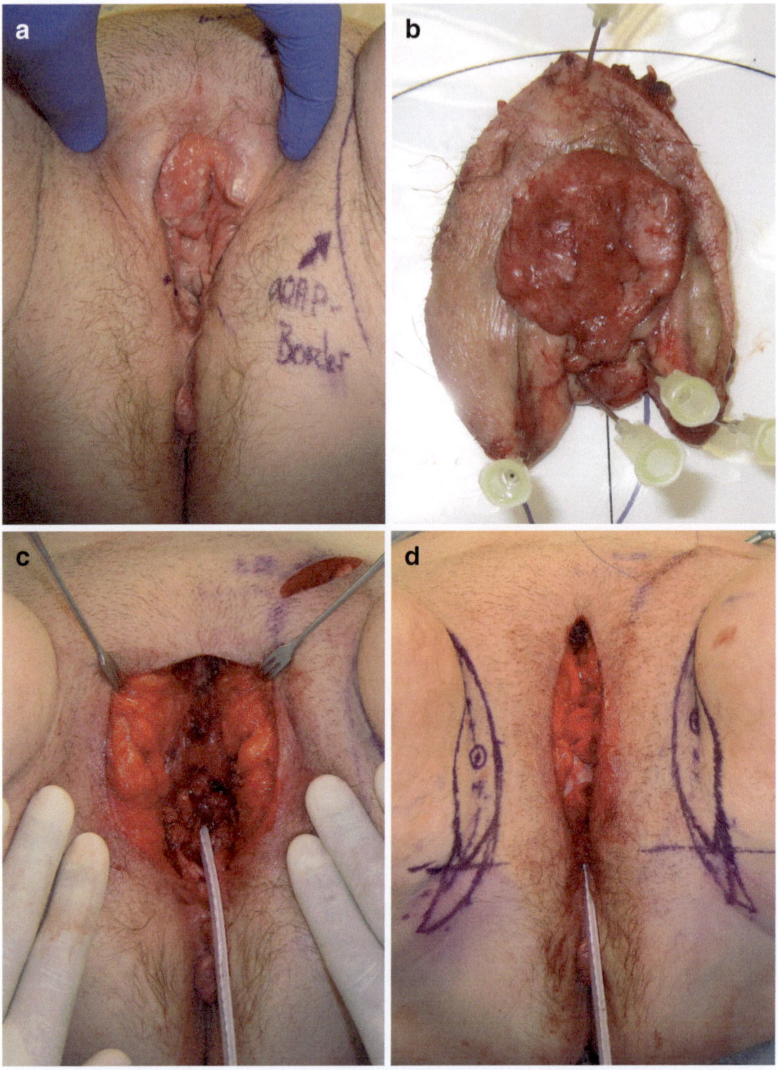

Fig. 1.14 60-Year-old woman with an extensive vulvar cancer of the anterior commissure including region of the clitoral tip. (**a**) (top left) Preoperative view showing extension of the tumor; medial border of the aOAP-flap incision line and placement of the inguinal incision are marked on the left side to realize topographic relations. (**b**) (top right) Intraoperative view after tumor excision including the region of the clitoral tip; tumor excision comprises inguinal lymph nodes of the left side not shown in this picture. (**c**) (middle left) Intraoperative view after excision of the tumor including excision of the clitoral tip showing extension of the defect; the clitoral stump located at the middle of the clitoral bodies is visible in the upper part of the defect. (**d**) (middle right) Intraoperative view after excision of the tumor and both sided planning of the aOAP flaps on the genitofemoral sulcus. (**e**) (bottom left) Intraoperative view after medially tunneled transposition of the both sided aOAP flaps and closure of the harvest side by means of a medial thigh lift. (**f**) (bottom right) Intraoperative view after complete aOAP-flap inset demonstrating flexibility of the reconstructed vaginal introitus and simultaneously reconstructed clitoral tip with NMCS procedure positioned 1.5 cm anterior to the urethral orifice

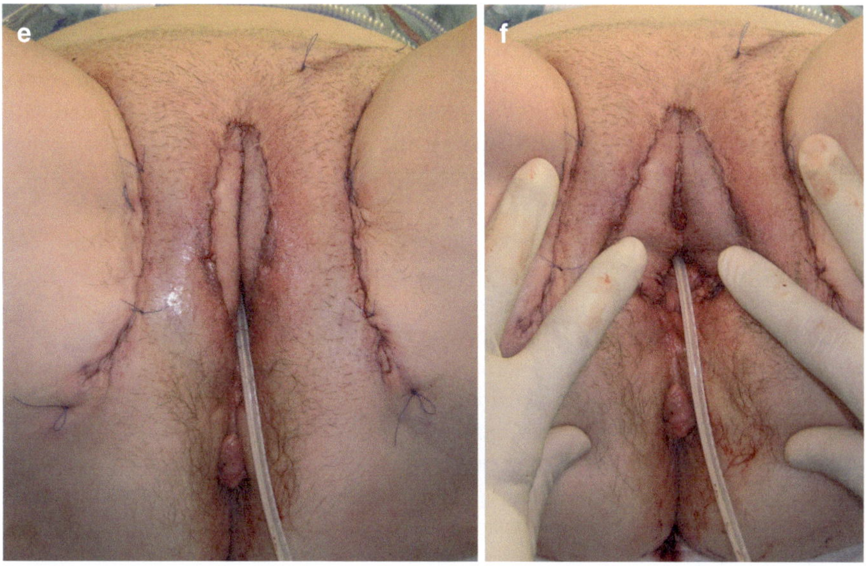

Fig. 14 (continued)

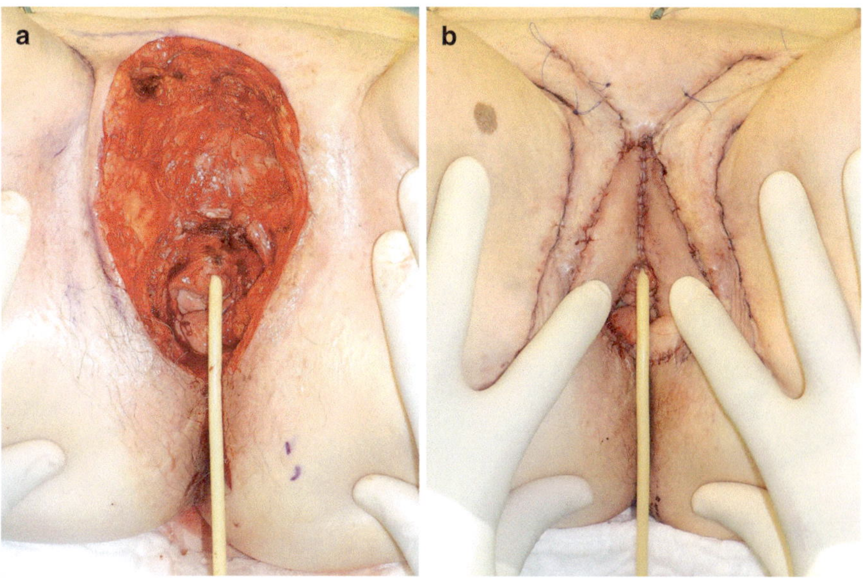

Fig. 1.15 77-Year-old woman with an extensive cancer of the vaginal introitus and the anterior commissure including region of the clitoris. (**a**) (left) Intraoperative view following wide excision including region of the clitoris and both sided inguinal lymph nodes. (**b**) (right) Immediate reconstructive result with both sided tunneled aOAP flaps for vulvar reconstruction, both sided medial thigh lift for closure of the harvest side, and an advancement-transposition flap of the mons; flexibility of the vaginal introitus is shown

Inflammation of the Bartholin glands is of particular importance involving almost 2% of all women [16]. The Bartholin glands are located at the 4 and 8 o'clock positions in the vestibule and drain both sides into it. Unfortunately they sometimes develop abscesses or cysts. Bartholin gland abscess in turn can be associated with phlegmonous cellulitis of the surrounding tissues. As with other abscesses, patients tend to apply pressure to the lesion in an attempt to initiate drainage and relief but potentially aggravate the inflammatory process.

Concerning surgical intervention, healing usually occurs after surgical relief, permanent draining by suturing the wall of the gland to the epidermis of the vestibule (marsupialization). Marsupialization usually cures the disease but may also result in symptomatic scarring, tissue depression with an open introitus, and dyspareunia. In addition, secondary sclerosis of the surrounding tissue and painful scarring may also occur leading to revisional operative interventions. Operative revision should be consequently more sustainable by means of radical excision and immediate reconstruction. The aOAP flap procedure shows many benefits for reconstruction of the perineal and bordering region. Due to flap mobility and tissue thickness of the aOAP flap molding of the posterior commissure and the perineum works very well (Fig. 1.16).

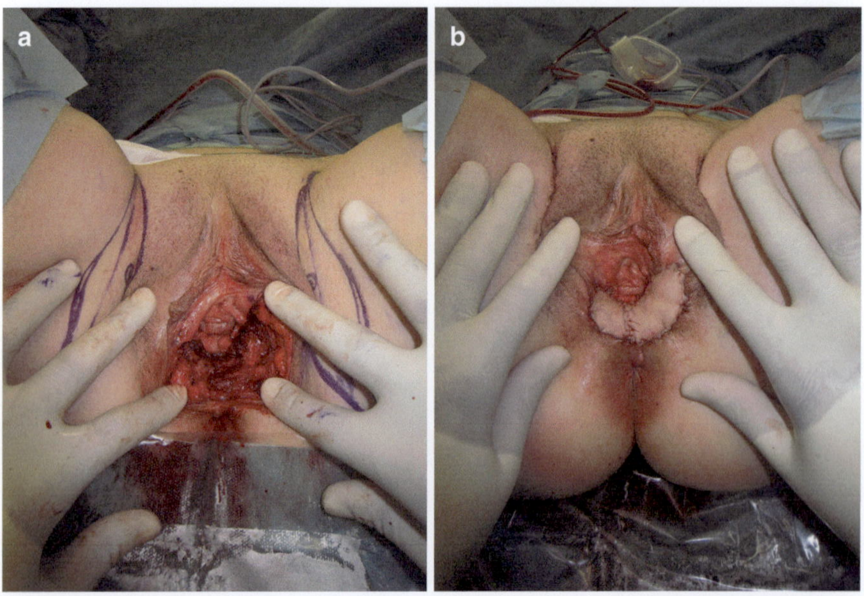

Fig. 1.16 50-Year-old woman with recurrent inflammation of the Bartholin glands; multiple operative interventions elsewhere were done; she presented with fibrous induration of the perineum, symptomatic scarring, and painful masses of the region of the Bartholin glands. (**a**) (left) Intraoperative view after both sided wide excision including the region of the perineum; the remaining three-dimensional defect requires an all-layered reconstruction. (**b**) (right) Immediate reconstruction with both sided tunneled aOAP flaps, and bilateral medial thigh lift for closure of the harvest side; flexibility of the posterior vaginal introitus is shown

1.6.4 Functional Disorders

The term "vulvodynia" represents a genital condition of chronic or acute pain and discomfort without evidence of inflammatory, infectious, neoplastic, nonneoplastic, or any other origin. As a result it is difficult to identify and even more difficult to handle. Symptoms can be triggered by mechanical stress like sexual intercourse or spontaneously. However, complaints should be taken seriously.

The symptomatic region can range from clearly defined areas to the entire vulva. Sometimes, in young patients a tight web at the posterior commissure, that does not tend to widen but tenses up through sexual intercourse, may cause the symptoms. A fine double-opposed Z-plasty, known as a dancing-man plasty, can solve the problem (Fig. 1.17a, b). Suturing of the flaps, however, must be performed meticulously in a multilayered fashion. I prefer resorbable suture material like monofilament 5.0 and 6.0 for subcutaneous sutures and braided 6.0 for skin closure in a single-knot fashion.

The therapeutic approach must be decided in the individual case and comprises treatment with ointments, symptomatic medications, nerve blocks, pain management, and psychosomatic or psychiatric approaches. In cases in which those conservative treatments are in the long run unsuccessful, surgery might be an option. In my experience partial vulvectomy and immediate anatomic reconstruction can lead to complete pain release (see Fig. 1.16). However, even though in selected cases a partial vulvectomy and anatomic reconstruction with the aOAP flap is a very effective procedure, it must be carefully considered because it is a complex

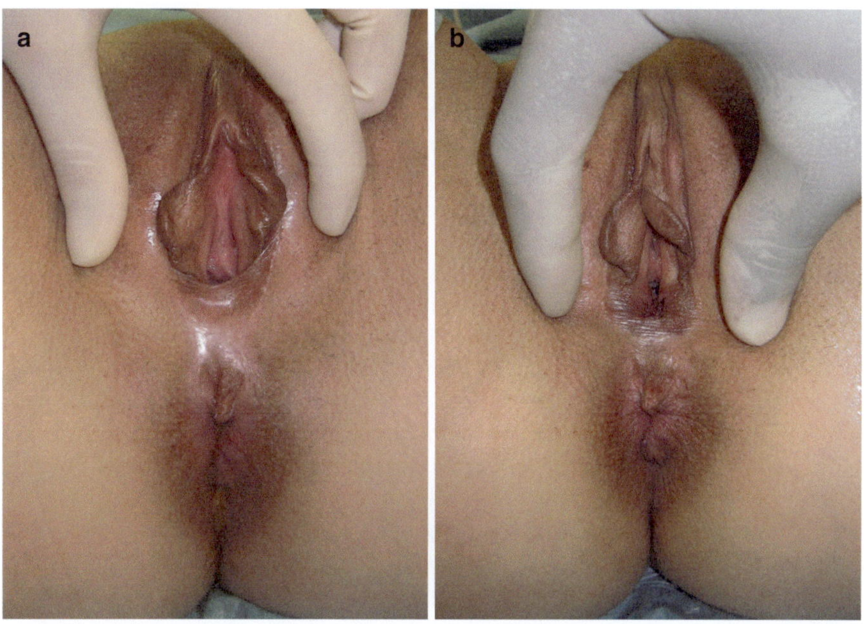

Fig. 1.17 26-year-old woman showing a symptomatious tight web at the posterior commissure; (**a**) (*left*) Preoperative view demonstrating the web while tighten up the posterior commissure. (**b**) (*right*) Postoperative view showing the faded web while tighten up the posterior commissure following a local dancing man plasty (opposed Zplasty)

intervention. Nevertheless, what cures cannot be wrong. Surgery, therefore, is an option especially in complex cases.

The term "dyspareunia" can be associated with "vulvodynia" but can in contrast also result from scarring based on diverse vulvar deformities. Women usually suffer from pain and discomfort triggered by sexual intercourse. Etiology is widespread including scarring resulting from FGM/C, diseases, traumas, or any operative intervention. Perineal lacerations and/or episiotomies do frequently induce chronic pain and may also be present with an open introitus leading into dryness and further problems. Relief can be achieved with local scar therapies using massages combined with ultrasonic technology and softening ointments. In conservative unsuccessful cases and in those in which a more complex deformity exists, scar excision and perineal reconstruction with the aOAP flap is an effective option (Fig. 1.18). The aOAP flaps can be used single sided just to fill in the preexisting tissue gap, or sided in an interlocking manner in the region of the perineum.

1.7 Justifying Indication for Reconstruction in FGM/C Patients

FGM/C is closely linked to tradition. Tradition is something very important for those people living with it, and that's why people need to carefully handle other people's traditions just to keep the intercultural communication and integrity of the respective culture. Respectful cultural interaction, however, does not mean unreflected acceptance of evident violation of human rights. Acceptance in that context means respectful interaction with those people being involved in certain traditions. From an intercultural point of view it might be beneficial and likewise advisable to call the practice of culturally motivated genital alterations "female genital cutting (FGC)" instead of "female genital mutilation (FGM)," just to respectfully reflect the cultural background of it. This is of course only a small differentiation but might have a major impact on the dignity and the cultural background of the patients. When at some point this context is understood, it will get clearer what great significance it has, that women search for reconstructive surgery, and what responsibility thereby is shouldered by the plastic or reconstructive surgeon. The term "mutilation" within the acronym "FGM," however, is a clear message outlining harm and injustice. It is a "must," therefore, to use both acronyms "FGM" and "FGC" individually in certain circumstances.

Regarding the cultural impact of FGM/C, who does justify reconstruction of the female genital in those patients? Should a woman be informed about her condition of being cut even though she might not be aware of it? Of course these are more philosophical than medical questions, but nevertheless important. When I was traveling through Tanzania in 2013, learning more about the roots of FGM/C, I quite rapidly came to the understanding that besides medical indication it must be of course the right of self-determination of both genders. Unfortunately,

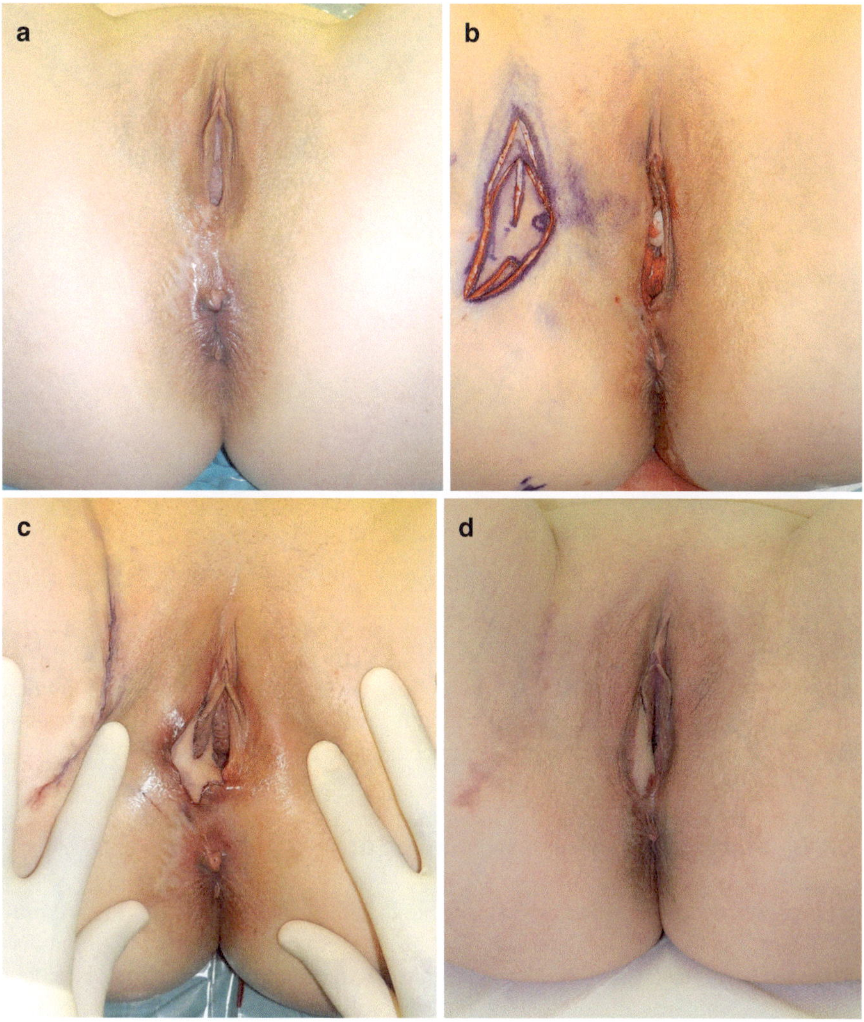

Fig. 1.18 30-Year-old woman with symptomatic scarring and dyspareunia after perineal laceration through delivery and episiotomy on the right side. (**a**) (top left) Preoperative view showing scarring of the posterior commissure and right-sided perineum. (**b**) (top right) Intraoperative view after scar excision as well as incision and tailoring of the aOAP flap to fill in the complex tissue defect. (**c**) (middle left) Intraoperative view after inset of the tailored aOAP flap on the right side. (**d**) (middle right) Frontal view 1 year postoperatively showing inconspicuous scarring of the vulva and the harvest side though there is a color mismatch concerning the aOAP flap and the vulva; nevertheless, preoperative complaints of the patient are gone. (**e**) (bottom left) Oblique view 1 year postoperatively showing more details of the three-dimensional aOAP-flap inset. (**f**) (bottom right) 1-Year follow-up examination in the upright position; note the normal contour of the vulva and inconspicuous scarring of the harvest side

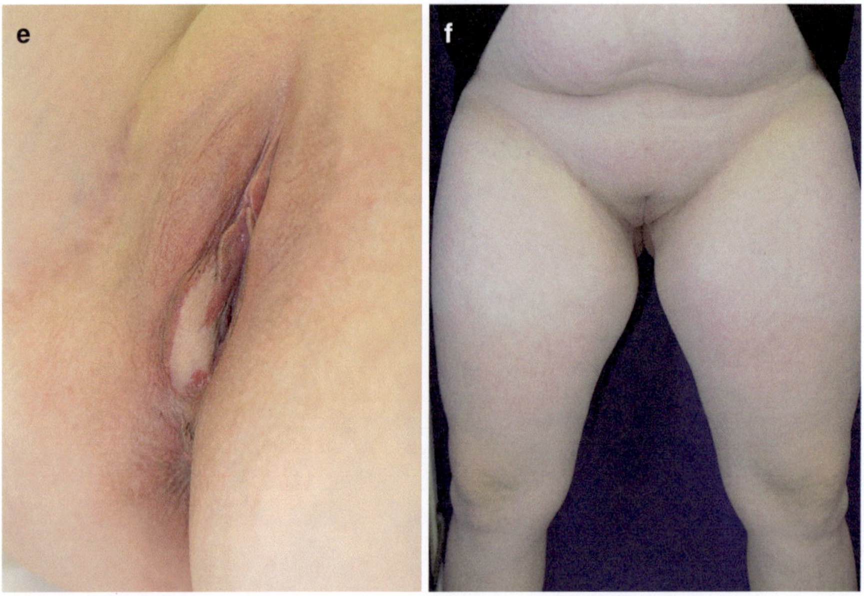

Fig. 18 (continued)

self-determination is not handled as a birth-given natural right of all human beings. Especially in women it is something, which is traditionally not prevalent in every country of the the world. That needs to be changed.

1.7.1 Importance of Reconstructive Surgery

Reconstructive surgery is the specialty able to return altered anatomy toward normal states. Besides physical damage FGM/C consequently leads to emotional distress that may last for a lifetime. Reconstructive surgery, therefore, is a key component in the interaction of all disciplines working together to end FGM/C. With some limitations, it can restore normal anatomy to bring back what was taken. This capacity is of an inestimable physical and psychological value for the affected. It is like establishing a solid fundament for all those things that need to be repaired. That is why most of my FGM/C patients report that they could at least begin a new life following reconstruction. Anatomic reconstruction is like the opening point of a restart.

Reconstruction, however, must be taken literally. There is a clear difference between the closure of an anatomic region that has a tissue deficit and the reconstruction of it (see Figs. 1.19, 1.20, and 1.21). From a reconstructive point of view, when comparing surgical results shown in Figs. 1.19, 1.20, and 1.21 it is obvious that the one performed with the combined pudendal thigh flap and gluteal VY-flap (Fig. 1.19) as well as the one with the gluteal VY-flaps only cannot compete with that one made with the aOAP flap (Fig. 1.21). It is clear that all those defects were

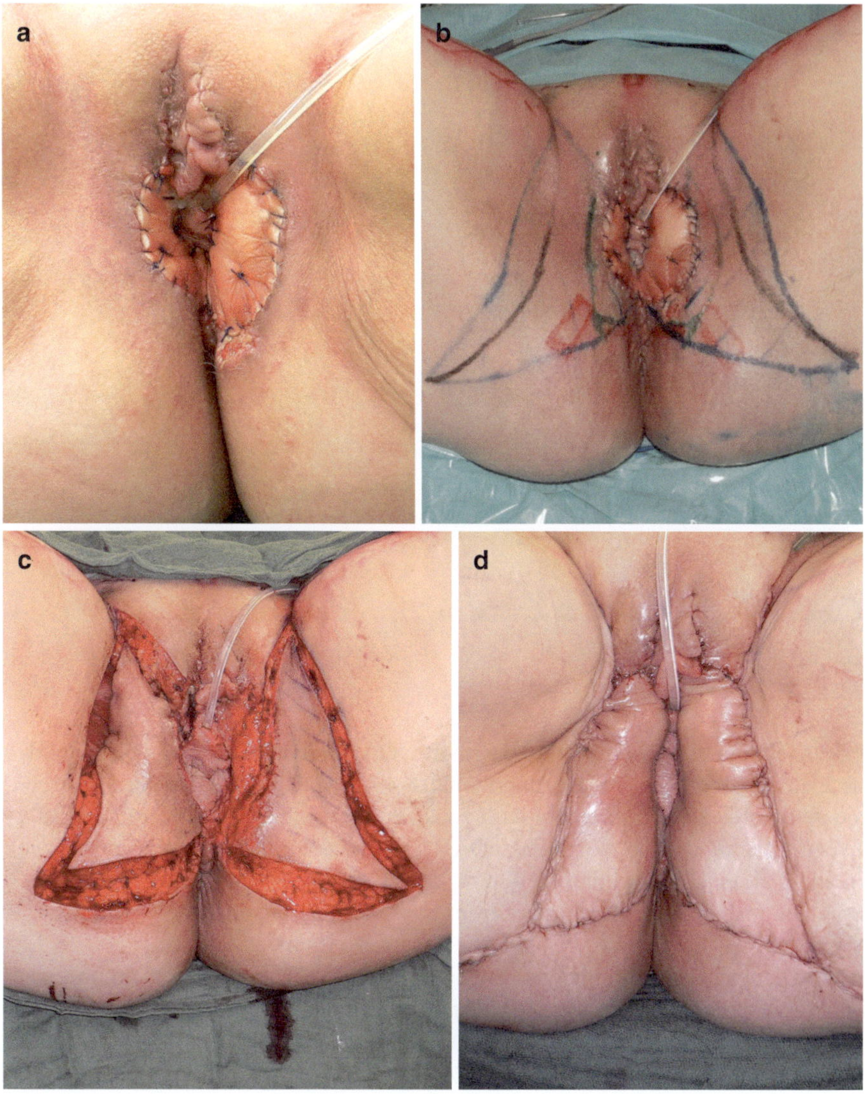

Fig. 1.19 52-Year-old woman showing an extensive defect of the posterior vulva and perineum after excision of a carcinoma; defect closure was planned and performed with a non-aOAP flap procedure by means of a pudendal thigh and gluteal VY-flap. (**a**) (top left) Preoperative view showing the vulvar defect covered with an alloplastic material as an interim solution; tumor excision and both sided inguinal lymph node dissection were performed beforehand; defect closure is intended secondary. (**b**) (top right) Intraoperative view showing planning for defect closure by means of a pudendal thigh flap combined with a both sided gluteal VY-flap. (**c**) (middle left) Intraoperative view after debridement of the vulvar defect and flap dissection. (**d**) (middle right) Intraoperative view after inset of the flaps; note that different aesthetic units are melt to one unit producing an artificial impression. (**e**) (bottom left) Frontal view 1 year postoperatively showing extended scarring of the vulva and the harvest side; nevertheless, wound closure was successful and stable. (**f**) (bottom right) 1-Year follow-up examination in the upright position; note the flattened contour of the vulva and conspicuous scarring

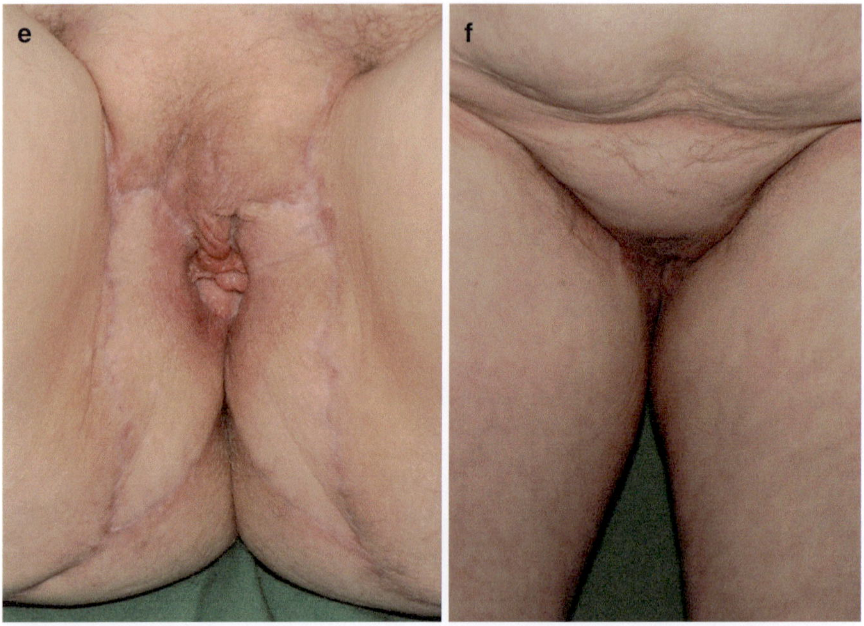

Fig. 19 (continued)

effectively closed, but only the one with the aOAP flap technique might be regarded as anatomically reconstructed. Important reconstructive aspects that need to be considered include replacing equal with equal, considering aesthetic units, and effectively reducing visible scars. The aOAP flap procedure for vulvar reconstruction includes all these claims and even more than that.

Regarding FGM/C the number of affected women is still rising. Actually it is estimated that the number of affected women is amounted to almost 200 million excluding a significant number of undetected victims. This leads into an important task for reconstructive surgeons all over the world and for other professionals dealing with the elimination of that problem. Partly or completely restoring anatomy of the vulva, however, is demanding due to the fact that FGM/C causes complex tissue loss. Techniques used for reconstruction must consider diverse morphologic details of normal anatomy including the excess and softness of labial tissue, the elasticity of the vaginal introitus, as well as the exposed position of the clitoral glans hooded by the clitoral prepuce. The reconstructive basis of all these factors will contribute to restore both an anatomically normal form and a normal function of the outer female genital likewise supporting psychophysical balance of the patients.

Concerning a natural reconstruction of the vulva including functional gain of the clitoris, the tunneled anterior obturator artery perforator flap (aOAP flap) invented and originally described by the author in 2010 [17]; the OD flap for prepuce reconstruction invented and originally described by the author in 2014 [18, 19]; and the NMCS procedure for microsurgical reconstruction of the clitoral tip invented by the

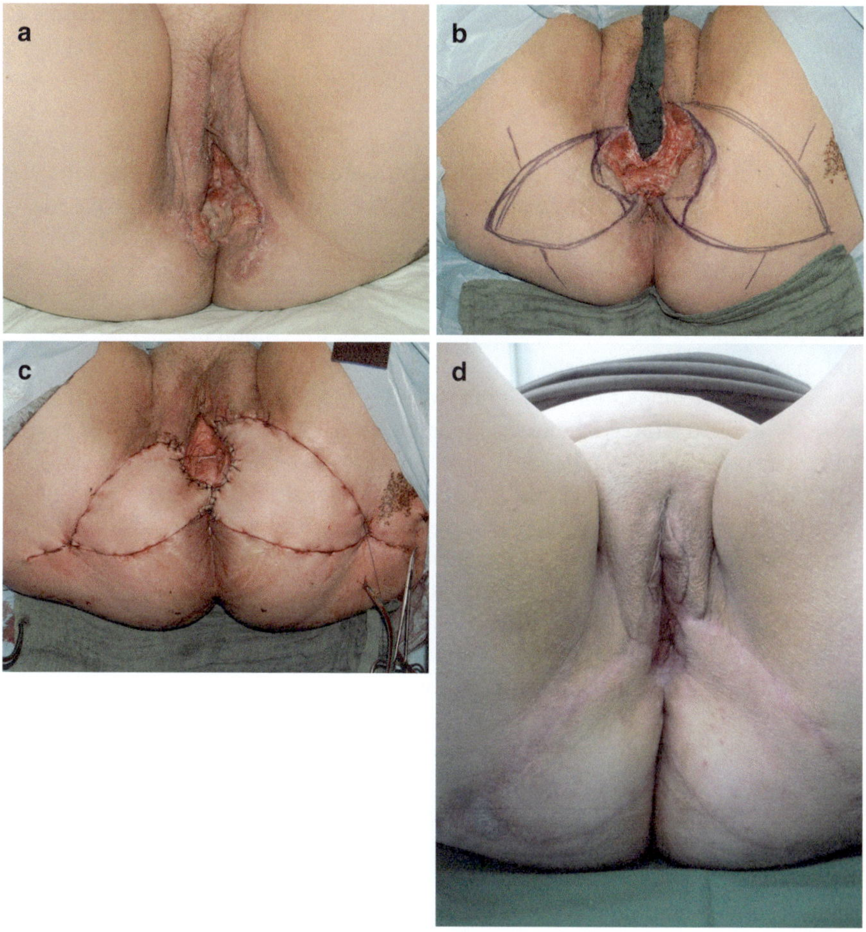

Fig. 1.20 43-Year-old woman showing an extensive defect of the posterior vulva and perineum after excision of a carcinoma; defect closure was planned and performed with a non-aOAP flap procedure by means of a gluteal VY-flap. (**a**) (top left) Preoperative view showing the vulvar defect; tumor excision and both sided inguinal lymph node dissection were performed beforehand; defect closure is intended secondary. (**b**) (top right) Intraoperative view showing planning for defect closure by means of a both sided gluteal VY-flap. (**c**) (bottom left) Intraoperative view after debridement of the vulvar defect, flap dissection, and transposition for defect closure; note that different aesthetic units are melt to one unit producing an artificial impression. (**d**) (bottom right) Frontal view 1 year postoperatively showing extended scarring of the vulva and the harvest side; posterior vulva shows a flattened contour; nevertheless, wound closure was successful and stable

author and originally described in 2017 [19] offer exceptional results. I presented these techniques for the first time on the 46th annual meeting of the German Society of Plastic, Reconstructive and Aesthetic Surgeons (DGPRÄC; Deutsche Gesellschaft der Plastischen, Rekonstruktiven und Ästhetischen Chirurgen) in 2015 in Berlin as part of a key lecture and a live surgery course performed on a young patient suffering from ablative surgery following vulvar cancer. All these procedures of mine proved to have natural, reliable, and long-lasting results while normalizing anatomy of the mutilated and/or deformed outer female genital.

1.7.2 Importance of Defibulation by Means of a Vulvar Opening Versus Vulvar Reconstruction in FGM/C Type III Patients

Well, sometimes decision-making in FGM/C patients is problematic. FGM/C type III, also known as "infibulation," means amputation of almost all parts of the outer genitalia including the prepuce, significant parts of the clitoral organ, minor labias, and major labias. The external orifice of the urethra and most of the vestibule is covered by adaptation of the remaining wound edges. The posterior-most part of the vestibule in the region of the posterior commissure is left open to enable passage of urine and menstrual blood. Passage, however, is restricted. As a result, the vagina is left largely inaccessible. Regular function of the clitoral organ is effectively destroyed by partly excision, suppressing potential sexual pleasure. The remaining clitoral organ is kept buried. In prevalent countries performing FGM/C type III reopening of the vulva called "defibulation" is routinely performed in different ways depending on tradition, namely, at the time of first "official" sexual intercourse. "Official" in that context means "generally accepted by the community." Re-infibulation following the successfully performed sexual act, however, is also routine in many places.

All around the world physicians are faced with patients suffering from distinct types of FGM/C. Especially those suffering from FGM/C type III frequently show significant physical damage and complaints. Moreover some of FGM/C type III patients simply ask for vulvar opening motivated by them or their husbands or sexual partners to improve or realize penetration. Vulvar opening only can reduce complaints and does improve vulvar function for both sexual and birth-related concerns [20, 21, 22]. From a reconstructive point of view, however, the result of "defibulation" only is clearly not equivalent to the effectiveness of complex vulvar reconstruction. That's why it should be justified to differentiate between an "*opening-defibulation*," meaning a single opening of the vulvar remnant, and "*reconstructive-defibulation*," meaning opening of the vulva followed by complex autologous restoration of that what's missing. Due to the benefits achieved by complex vulvar reconstruction with the described techniques, reconstructive-defibulation should be made available not only in individual cases, because it is the latest and likewise most effective way existing today able to restore vulvar anatomy.

Why shouldn't we adapt specialized techniques enabling us to offer the latest achievements in vulvar reconstruction to FGM/C patients even though we could? The anatomic resultant of FGM/C or other acquired deformities—that is, major tissue loss—opposes the same reconstructive demands for example as after ablative breast procedures. Nobody will deny that autologous breast reconstruction evolved as the gold standard in reconstructive breast surgery even though microsurgical tissue transfer is complex, time consuming, and not an "everybody's procedure."

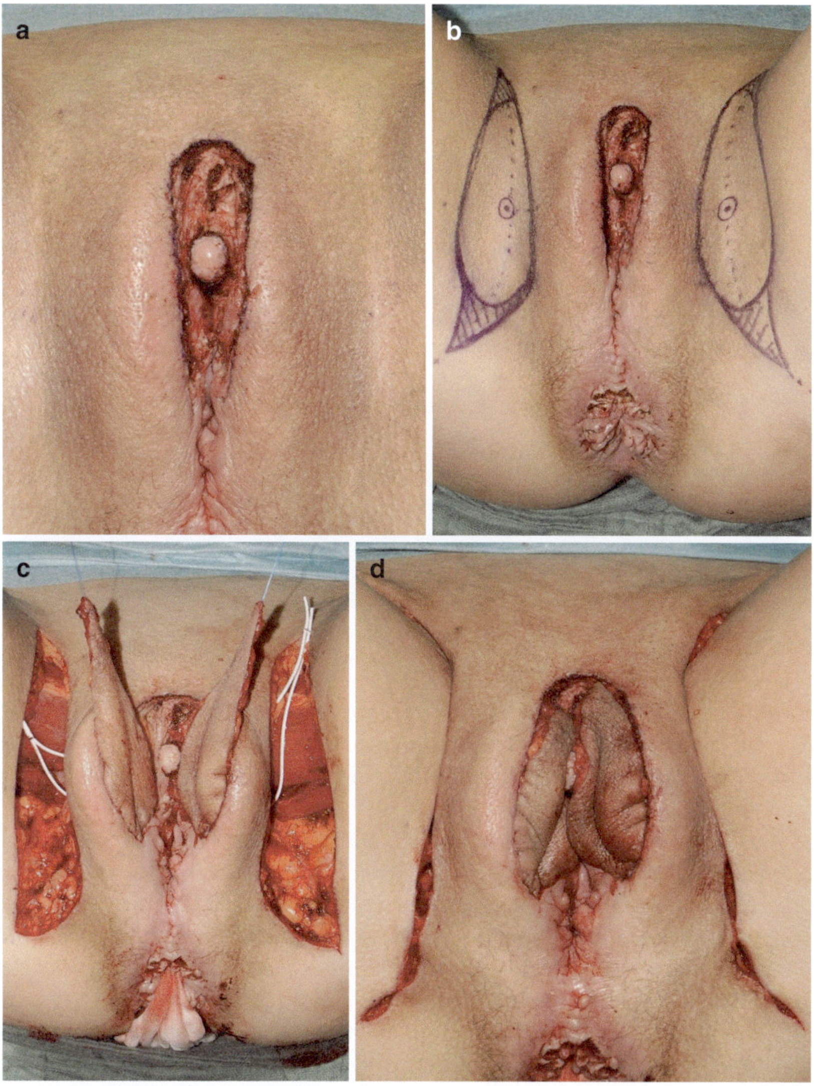

Fig. 1.21 29-Year-old woman showing an extensive defect of the vulva after excision of a neoplasia; defect closure was planned and performed with the tunneled, both sided aOAP flap procedure. (**a**) (top left) Intraoperative view showing the vulvar defect; tumor excision was performed beforehand; defect closure is performed primarily. (**b**) (top right) Intraoperative view showing planning for reconstruction by means of a both sided, tunneled aOAP flap; flap dimensions are outlined including position of the perforator vessel placed eccentrically at the medial border of both flaps in line with the genitofemoral sulcus. (**c**) (middle left) Intraoperative view after flap harvesting and tunneled transpositioning into the vulvar defect. (**d**) (middle right) Intraoperative view after inset of the flaps; note the floppy and soft issue of both flaps arranged as an aesthetic unit. (**e**) (bottom left) Frontal view 1 year postoperatively showing a natural aspect of the vulva, being reconstructed as an aesthetic unit; note the inconspicuous scarring of the vulva and the harvest side. (**f**) (bottom right) 1-Year follow-up examination in the upright position; note the natural contour of the vulva and conspicuous scarring

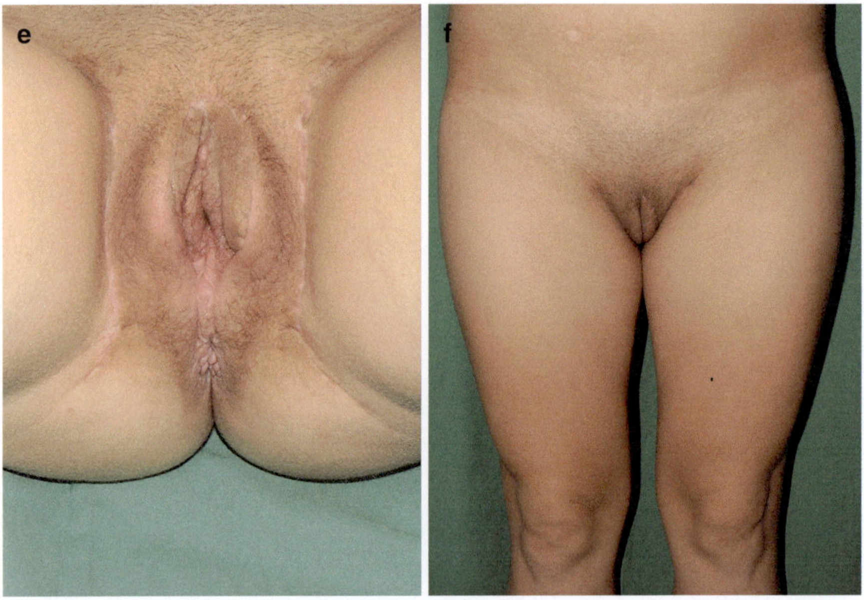

Fig. 21 (continued)

However, concerning medical progress we need to orientate on such benchmarks to refine our standards. Generally, patients all over the world should be offered to benefit from the latest achievements in medicine even though it must be tailored to the respective healthcare structure.

Again, anatomically, the main problem with FGM type III is the major tissue loss followed by subtotal closure of the vulva, all of which lead into reduced elastic capacity of the remaining vulva aggravated by tension and scarring, and loss of vulvar function due to deformation. Vulvar opening only does not add any tissue and therefore does not solve every anatomic problem associated with infibulation. The main advantages of single vulvar opening are the improvement of micturition, menstruation, and hygiene, as well as enabling for penetration (Fig. 1.22). Capacity of vaginal delivery, however, is debatable following vulvar opening only, because there is still significant tension and restrictive elasticity in the region of the middle and the anterior vulva or the anterior commissure, respectively. It is advisable, therefore, to critically evaluate the outer genital prior to delivery [23]. If the risk of serious tissue damage possibly forced by vaginal delivery is deemed too high, cesarean section should be considered. Complex vulvar reconstruction, then, can and should be reflected secondarily, in particular because vaginal delivery should almost always be enabled through aOAP-flap reconstruction in FGM type III patients.

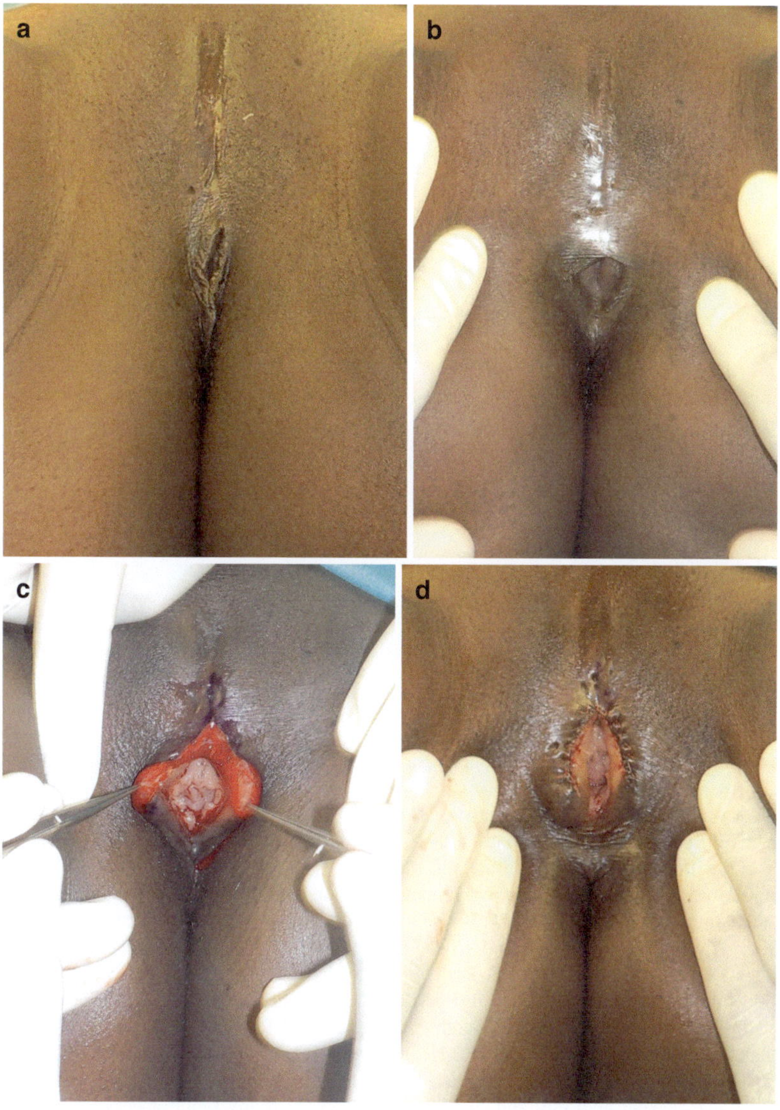

Fig. 1.22 28-Year-old woman showing a type III genital cutting (infibulation) with amputated prepuce, clitoral tip and body, minor, and major labias that are adapted to a narrowed vaginal opening. (**a**) (top left) Preoperative view showing the vulva at rest. (**b**) (top right) Preoperative view showing the vulva at slight tension; note the narrowed vaginal opening and the restricted skin elasticity due to tissue loss by amputation. (**c**) (middle left) Intraoperative view after surgical separation by a simple cut through the middle ("deinfibulation"); cut edges are held with fine forceps; care should be taken to limit the anterior cut edge to the border of the anterior vestibulum. (**d**) (middle right) Intraoperative view after wound closure on both sides; closure should be performed in two layers with fine and resorbable suture material (e.g., monofilament resorbable 6.0 subcutaneously and braided resorbable 6.0 cutaneously); note that there is still no gain of elasticity besides and anterior to the recreated opening. (**e**) (bottom left) Postoperative view at rest 1 year after vulvar opening; elasticity of the vestibule and the anterior vulva is still lacking. (**f**) (bottom right) Postoperative view in the upright position; contour of the vulva is normal

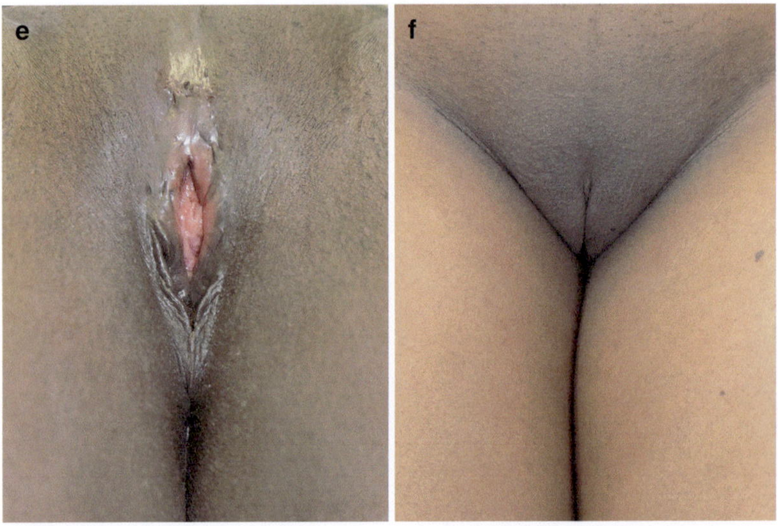

Fig. 22 (continued)

Literature

1. World Health Organization. Eliminating female genital mutilation: an interagency statement. Geneva: World Health Organization, Department of Reproductive Health and Research; 2008. p. 1–48.
2. O'Connell HE, Sanjeevan KV, Hutson J. Anatomy of the clitoris. J Urol. 2005;174:1189–95.
3. UNICEF. Female genital mutilation. 2016. http://www.unicef.org/media/files/FGMC_2016_brochure_final_UNICEF_SPREAD.pdf
4. European Parliament. European parliament resolution of 24 March 2009 on combating female genital mutilation in the EU (2008/2071(INI)). 2009. http://www.europarl.europa.eu/sides/getDoc.do?pubRef=//EP//NONSGML+TA+P6-TA-2009-0161+0+DOC+PDF+Vo//EN
5. Mack-Detlefsen B, Banaschak S, Boemers TM. Traumatic vulvar epithelial inclusion cysts following female genital mutilation (FGM). Geburtshilfe Frauenheilkd. 2015;75(9):945–8.
6. WHO. A systemic review of the health complications of female genital mutilation including sequelae in childbirth. Geneva: World Health Organization; 2000. p. 1–81.
7. Abdulcadir J, Botsikas D, Bolmont M, Bilancioni A, Djema DA, Demicheli FB, Yaron M, Petignat P. Sexual anatomy and function in women with and without genital mutilation: a cross-sectional study. J Sex Med. 2016;13(2):226–37.
8. Meffert JJ, Davis BM, Grimwood RE. Lichen sclerosus. J Am Acad Dermatol. 1995;32:393–416.
9. Burger MPM, Obdeijn MC. Complications after surgery for the relief of dyspareunia in women with lichen sclerosus: a case series. Acta Obstet Gynecol Scand. 2016;95:467–72.
10. Neil SM, Lewis FM, Tatnall FM, Cox NH. British Association of Dermatologists' guidelines for the management of lichen sclerosus. Br J Dermatol. 2010;63:672–82.
11. Bradford J, Fischer G. Surgical division of labial adhesions in vulvar lichen sclerosus and lichen planus. J Low Genit Tract Dis. 2013;17:48–50.
12. Lee A, Bradford J, Fischer G. Long-term management of adult vulvar lichen sclerosus. A prospective cohort study of 507 women. JAMA Dermatol. 2015;151:1061–7.
13. Höckel H, Dornhöfer N. Vulvovaginal reconstruction for neoplastic disease. Lancet Oncol. 2008;9:559–68.

14. Sideri M, Jones RW, Wilkinson EJ, Preti M, Heller DS, Scurry J, Haefner H, Neill S. Squamous vulvar intraepithelial neoplasia. 2004 Modified terminology, ISSVD Vulvar Oncology Subcommitee. J Reprod Med. 2005;*50*:*807*–10.
15. Faro S. Infections of the vulva, vagina, and cervix. In: Kovac SR, Zimmermann CW, editors. Advances in reconstructive vaginal surgery, vol. 2007. Philadelphia: Wolters Kluwer/Lippincott Williams & Wilkins; 2007. p. 383–96.
16. Stenchever MA, Mishell D, Herbst A. Infections of the lower genital tract. Comprehensive gynecology. St Louis: Mosby; 2001. p. 482–6.
17. O'Dey DM, Bozkurt A, Pallua N. The anterior Obturator Artery Perforator (aOAP) flap: surgical anatomy and application of a method for vulvar reconstruction. Gynecol Oncol. 2010;119:526–30. Epub 2010 Sep 24.
18. O'Dey DM. Die rituelle Beschneidung der Klitorisregion: Anatomie und Wiederherstellung mittels Omega-Domed flap. Plast Chir. 2014;14(1):44–7.
19. O'Dey DM. Complex reconstruction of the vulva following female genital mutilation/cutting. Urologe. 2017;56(10):1298–301.
20. Johnson C, Nour NM. Surgical techniques: defibulation of Type III female genital cutting. J Sex Med. 2007;4:1544–7.
21. Seifeldin A. Genital reconstruction surgery after female genital mutilation. Obstet Gynecol Int J. 2016;4(6):00129. https://doi.org/10.15406/ogij.201604.00129.
22. Madzou S, Ouédraogo CMR, Gillard P, Lefebvre-Lacoeuille C, Catala L, Sentilhes L, Descamps P. Chirurgie plastique reconstructice du clitoris après mutilations sexuelles. Ann Chir Plast Esthet. 2001;56:59–64.
23. O'Dey DM. Rekonstruktion nach ritueller Beschneidung. Deutsche Hebammenzeitschrift. 2014;12:51–4.

Basic Consideration

2

2.1 Clinical Setting

An optimal clinical setting for complex vulvar reconstruction should meet the requirements necessary for inpatient treatment. The facility must be specialized and well equipped, with well-qualified and motivated staff members, because therapy of FGM/C patients needs professionalism, accuracy, and passion. The facility should offer a pleasant examination room with a changing area, so that the patient can feel comfortable. Furthermore, a system to perform standardized photography should be available. Photographs, of course, are especially necessary to document the preoperative and postoperative status. The office-photography arrangement should provide two frontal light units for uniform illumination and a simple homogeneous background for increased contrast and reduced distraction to get photographs in the upright position (Fig. 2.1a). An examination chair should also be provided for office photography (Fig. 2.1b). Basic viewpoints include frontal (Fig. 2.1c) and back (Fig. 2.1d) while standing, as well as frontal with the vulva at rest (Fig. 2.1e) as well as the vulva slightly tightened (Fig. 2.1f) in the supine position with angled legs or the lithotomy position, respectively. The patient must be informed of and consent to the purpose of medical use of the photographs as well as electronic archiving of the personal data.

The surgeon requires in-depth understanding of anatomy of the female genital, and must be confident with the topography, and techniques of dissection under normal and changed anatomic conditions. The responsible surgeon with the help of a preferable female assistant should almost always perform the examination. In addition, a representative with translational skills or a translator should attend the examination from a separate area or at least attend the final talk. It should be guaranteed that the patient is overall informed about the prevailing anatomic condition, intended reconstruction, expectable improvement resulting from the operation, need for temporary bladder catheterization, postoperative care, delayed restart of sexual activity, temporary incapacity for work, and some more.

D. m. O´Dey, *Vulvar Reconstruction Following Female Genital Mutilation/Cutting (FGM/C) and other Acquired Deformities*,
https://doi.org/10.1007/978-3-030-02168-9_2

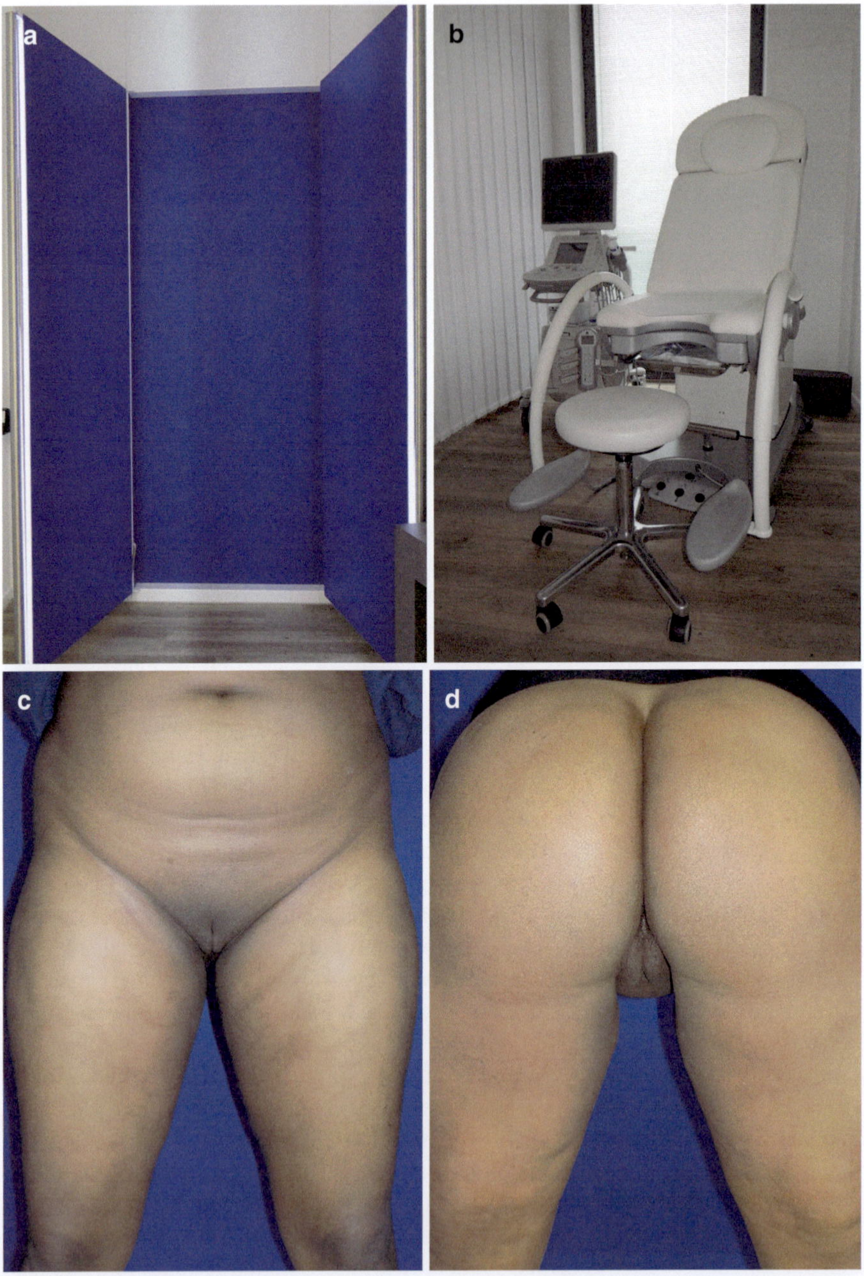

Fig. 2.1 Office photography. (**a**) (top left) Upright photography with a simple single-colored background. (**b**) (top right) Chair with angled legs for examination and photography. (**c**) (middle left) Standard upright position frontal view in a 27-year-old FGM/C III patient. (**d**) (middle right) Same patient standard upright position in back view (in cases following or scheduled for full vulvar reconstruction). (**e**) (bottom left) Same patient standard lithotomy position vulva at rest. (**f**) (bottom right) Same patient standard lithotomy position with the vulva slightly tightened up giving view to the vaginal introitus

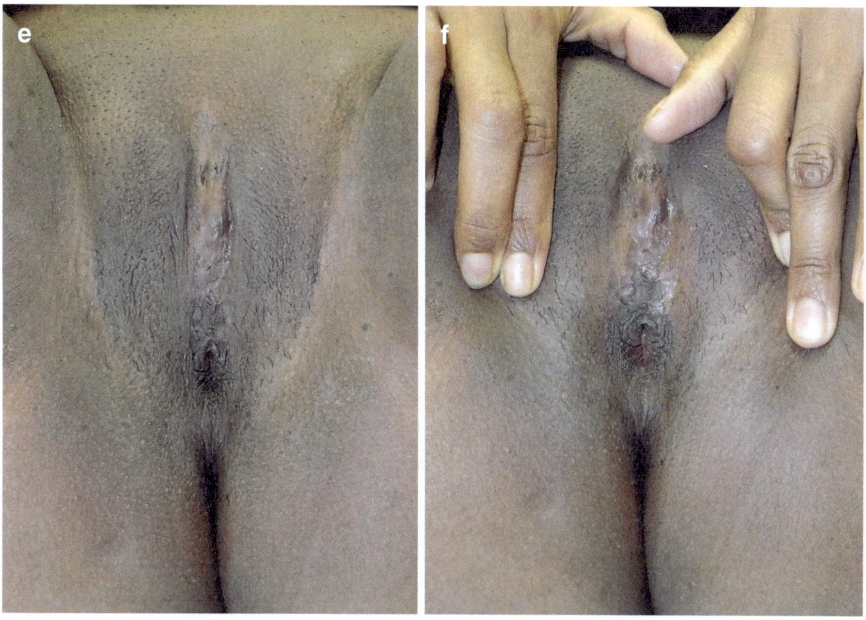

Fig. 2.1 (continued)

2.2 Patient Management

The vulva is a unique anatomic region and has a special significance for each individual. Concerning examination, the physician requires both an appropriate handling of and empathy for the patient. A profound review of the history is critical. FGM patients frequently do not dare to describe their problems clearly because they culturally used to not complain. On request, however, patients especially describe the occurrence of pain during menstruation, and sexual intercourse, as well as the absence of sexual sensation, and some more. In some patients inspection might be more appropriately performed in the operating room with the patient sedated or asleep. It is self-evident that every examination no matter where must be performed in consent with the patient. As mentioned above it is usually beneficial to have a representative accompanying the patient. It is important to find out what was done before. Interview, inspection, and palpation, therefore, are critical in examining the outer female genital. Inspection leads into an analytic overview of the underlying problem and the necessary reconstructive needs. The examiner gets an impression about the aOAP-flap harvest side at the thigh creases lateral to the vulva, pubic hair important for flap design or adjunctive procedures like epilation, and which parts of the vulva can be included in the reconstructive plan. It's enormous which information you get from adherence or sliding capacity of the overlying tissue or a scar to the underlying layers. Palpation of the inferior pubic ramus and the medial border of the obturator foramen half the way from the pubic body to the ischial tuberosity determine the aOAP vessel. Furthermore, palpation of the tissue overlying the symphysis brings information about the position of the remaining clitoral organ, existence of a clitoral cyst, or the symmetry pattern of the remaining skin. All the findings must then be correlated with the operative plan.

Patient management does further include optimizing operative and postoperative conditions. Preoperative mechanical bowel preparation using light magnesium oxide with citric acid and postoperative control of defecation should avoid contamination of the suture lines likewise reducing the risk of infection, wound-healing disorders, or flap lost. In addition, prophylactic antibiotics are administered intravenously on the day of surgery (Table 2.1) and up to two days after, followed by oral application for further 5 to 7 days postoperatively depending on the circumstances; painkillers and decongestive medication are applied for 5–8 days. In addition, some cases may profit from oral or systemic application of cortisone to reduce inflammatory response and swelling.

Especially in obese patients pressure relief at the flap site especially in region of the posterior commissure through angled legs on pillows in the supine position combined with pressure-reduced bedding is beneficial for 3–5 days until complete flap autonomy and reliable load capacity should have been achieved. During that time the patient is advised to stay in bed for 2 days postoperatively. I use to mobilize my patients out of bed on day 3 after surgery. Beforehand careful physiotherapy is performed in bed without impairing the operative result. The patient is further instructed in the use of the recommended ointments. The latter include an antibiotic ointment for outer suture lines, estrogen ointment for the region of the clitoris and the vaginal introitus, and heparin ointment in case of discoloration caused by superficial hematomas.

2.3 Clinical Management

FGM/C is a sensitive issue and patients are also. Clinical management, therefore, is complex. Once infrastructure is formed and specialized protocols have been well established, clinical management becomes easier. Beforehand, however, education is obligatory. All the staff members and nurses must be profoundly briefed about FGM/C itself. They should know about what generally happened to the patients, what kind of deformities exist, the need and importance of reconstructive surgery, the potential of reconstructive surgery, the advantage of up-to-date reconstructive procedures, and especially the postoperative care necessary to carry the patients to an overall successful result. This also includes empathy for cultural background of the patients. Sometimes FGM/C patients do not only feel satisfaction after surgery, but also undergo flashbacks of their childhood; that means flashbacks of FGM/C. It is therefore important to sensitize employees about possible psychological distress of the patients that should never ever be trivialized. Psychological adjunctive therapy therefore is an important option and sometimes necessary, but need to be

Table 2.1 Prophylactic antibiotics following vulvar reconstruction

Antibiotic	Concentration [g]	Application (intravenous)
Clindamycin	0.6	1-1-1
Cefuroxime	1.5	1-1-1
Metronidazole	0.5	1-0-1

decided in the individual case. Confronting each patient with psychological help will not find generally acceptance and is moreover not necessary. However, psychological help should not be underestimated especially in those patients unspecifically searching for help. FGM/C patients finding my office usually had had professional or unprofessional psychological support beforehand; it depends individually on whether such support should be continued or not. The will for reconstruction is usually strong in most of my patients, and the postoperative gain of form and function does not usually cause psychological instability but the very opposite.

2.4 Anatomy

All the following anatomic orientations refer to the dorsal lithotomy position and are modeled after standardized descriptions of the female genital. Anterior directs toward the mons pubis, and posterior directs toward the anus. Inferior means directed to the surgeon sitting in front of the patient. Superior directs toward the promontory of the sacrum. Lateral and medial depend on the sagittal plane, which divides the pelvic bone into halves in the superior-inferior view.

Anatomic descriptions given in the following are oriented toward the reconstructive needs and do not intend to give an overall overview of the female genital and bordering regions. Generally, the region anterior to the anus bordered by inferior rami of the pubic bones and the symphysis is called the urogenital region. Within that region the pudendal region comprises the outer female genital. The region below the urogenital region is called the anal region. The connecting region between the urogenital region and the anal region is called the perineum [1].

2.4.1 Region of the Clitoris

Personal anatomic dissections are highly recommended to train and improve the own surgical understanding and skills. Especially altered topographic conditions forced by former interventions such as genital mutilations assume that the surgeon is confident with the regular anatomy (Fig. 2.2). Besides morphologic conditions knowledge of vascular anatomy is imperative (Fig. 2.2b).

Anatomy of the clitoris is complex [2]. Interactive sexual function of the clitoral region including the clitoral organ (crura, body, glans), bulbs, distal urethra, and inferior vagina seems to be till date somewhat unclear [3, 4, 5]. The whole region seems to be in sum responsible for sexual function and orgasm [3]. The clitoral organ consists of an inner hidden and an outer visible part. The inner part is formed by the clitoral crura whereas the clitoral body terminated by the clitoral glans forms the outer part. The crura run parallel to the ischiopubic ramus while further advancing to the pubic symphysis to merge into the clitoral body [4, 5]. The clitoral crura thereby are geniculately curved and change their upward direction into a downward course of the clitoral bodies (Fig. 2.3a–f). The clitoral bodies are fixed to the symphysis by the suspensory ligament consisting of a superficial and a deep part [3, 6]. Due to their retraction force, both components of the suspensory ligament must be

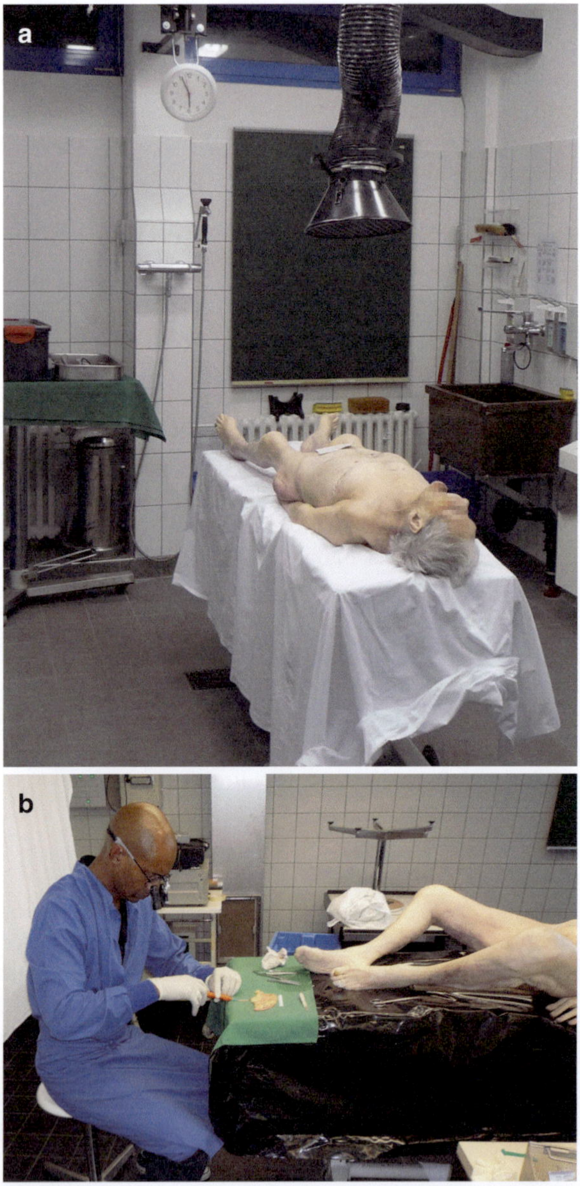

Fig. 2.2 Setting for anatomic dissections. (**a**) (top) Usual dorsal positioning of the corpse for anatomic dissection of the vulvar and inguinal region. (**b**) (bottom) Secondary vessel injection technique for further dissection of the vascular tree

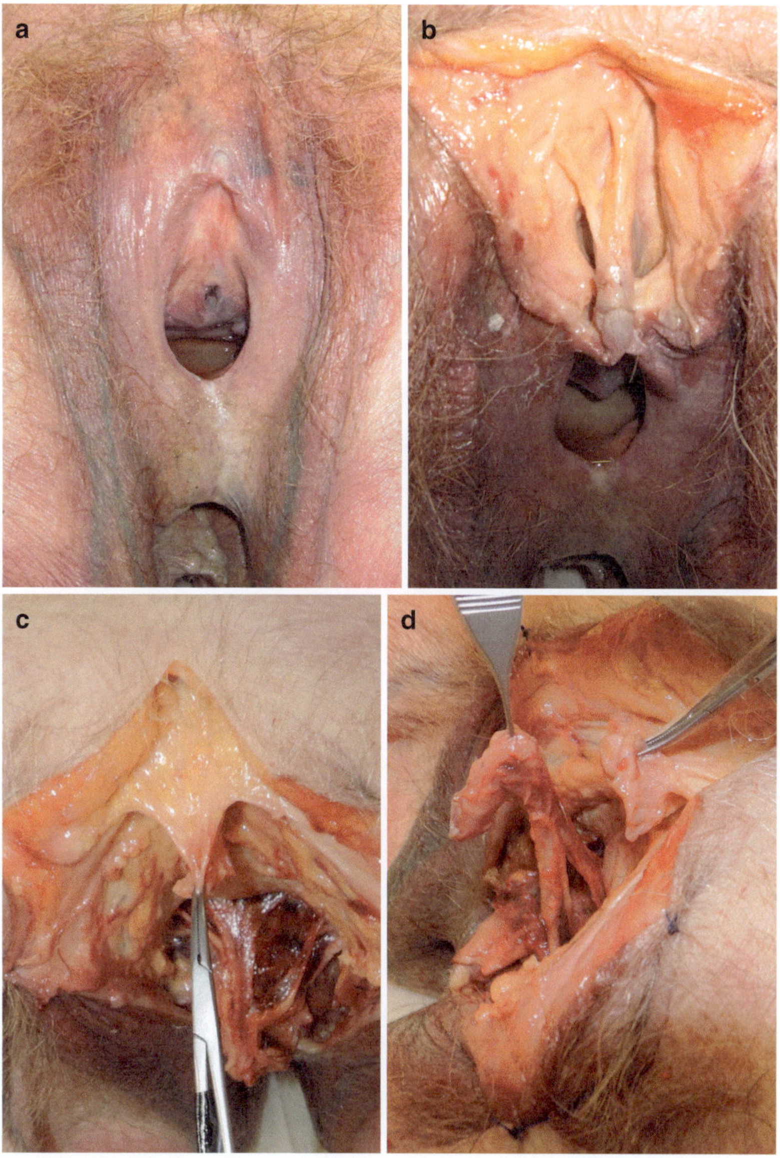

Fig. 2.3 Anatomic dissection detailing region of the clitoris in a 76-year-old corpse. (**a**) (top left) View of the outer female genital prior to dissection. (**b**) (top right) Anterior view of the clitoral organ after en bloc dissection with the clitoral tip and clitoral bodies as well as the superficial part of the suspensory ligament. (**c**) (middle left) Anterior view of the superficial part of the suspensory ligament (clamp) following separation from the clitoral organ. (**d**) (middle right) Lateral view showing the clitoral tip, clitoral bodies, and clitoral crura freed from the superficial and deep part of the suspensory ligament. (**e**) (bottom left) Ventral view of the clitoral organ; topography of the aOAP-perforator vessel close to the clitoral crura (marked with a yellow background on the left side, lateral to the inferior ramus of the pubic bone). (**f**) (bottom right) Dorsal view of the clitoral organ; topography of the clitoral nerves (marked with a yellow background) next to the clitoral artery and accompanying veins

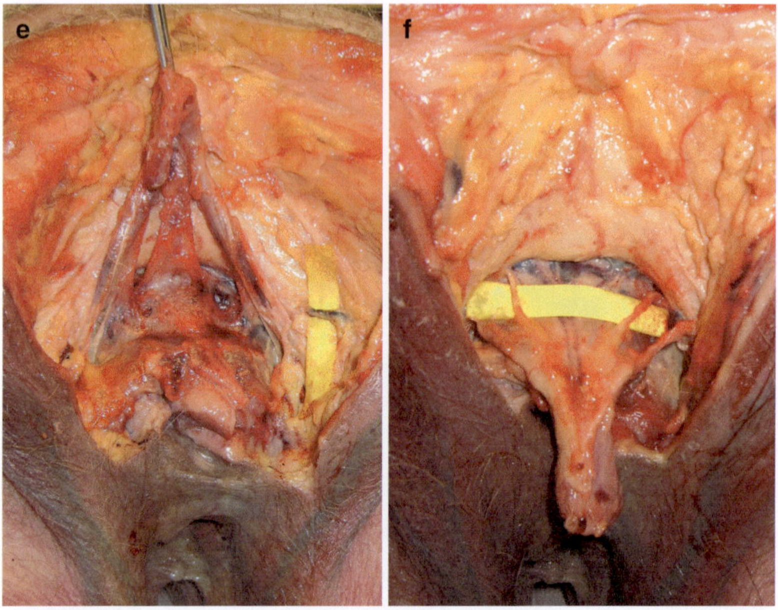

Fig. 2.3 (continued)

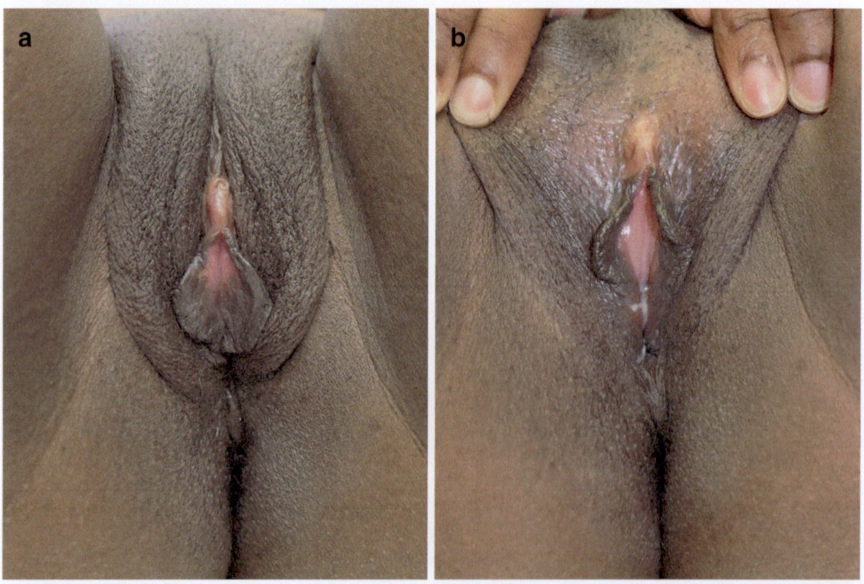

Fig. 2.4 Normally configured vulva of a 19-year-old woman. (**a**) (left) The normally configured vulva comprises (description from inside to outside): the vestibule in front of the hymen and the vaginal introitus being covered and flanked by the minor labias laterally, the clitoral tip anteriorly, and the perineum posteriorly; the minor labias are continued by the frenulum (roots of the minor labias) anteriorly followed by the clitoral prepuce; the major labias border the minor labias laterally. (**b**) (right) The normally configured vulva under slight lateral tension opening the vulvar vestibule

cut to the bone when mobilizing the retracted and straightened clitoral bodies during reconstruction (Fig. 2.3c, d). The clitoral bodies coalesce and terminate in the clitoral glans (Fig. 2.3b). That's why the clitoral bodies are almost always involved within the ritual of clitoral cutting.

In the normally configured, unimpaired vulva (Fig. 2.4) the clitoral prepuce covers both the visible part of the clitoris that means the clitoral glans and the upper invisible part that means the clitoral bodies. The posterior prepuce covering the clitoral glans thereby forms a hood, whereas the anterior part forms an anteriorly fading wall. The lower part of the prepuce merges into the minor labia, called "roots of the minor labias" (frenulum clitoridis). The split roots of the minor labias border the clitoral tip. The hoof-shaped space between the prepuce and the clitoral glans is called the coronary sulcus of the glans [1].

The pudendal plexus, originating from the second to fourth sacral segment of the spinal cord, is responsible for sensory supply of the clitoris [3, 5]. Branches course through the infrapiriform foramen directed to the symphysis. In region of the symphysis they form the dorsal clitoral branches innervating both the clitoral body and the clitoral glans (Fig. 2.3f). They travel along the upper surface of the clitoral body in the 11 and 1 o'clock positions [4] to finally enter the clitoral glans [3]. Within the glans both nerves spread into their terminal branches.

In FGM/C patients stumps of the clitoral nerves flanking the stump of the clitoral bodies need to be neurolysed microsurgically to make them eligible for successful reinnervation of the newly formed clitoral tip. That means that they need to be cut on a level showing healthy normally structured tissue. Detected neuromas, fibrous tissue, and scars must be excised.

2.4.2 Region of the Minor and Major Labias

Normal anatomy of the vulva is complex and unique (Fig. 2.4). The usually bulgy major labias border the pudendal column (rima pudenda), start at the anterior commissure, and end at the posterior commissure localized at the anterior border of the perineum. They contain fatty tissue traversed by a loose network of connective tissue bands. They show all over sebaceous as well as sweat glands and hair growth as part of the pubic hair. Between the major and the minor labias the interlabial sulcus is formed fading at the anterior and posterior commissure [1].

The minor labias run from the clitoral frenulum downward and mostly disappear on the level of the lower third of the flanking major labias or end within the frenulum labiorum pudendi at the posterior commissure. Due to the lacking fat layer, the minor labias are very narrow, filled with connective tissue showing sebaceous glands, and a rich vasculature including numerous veins. They do clearly vary in size and texture [7]. The opening between the minor labias is known as the vestibule. Within the vestibule and below the clitoral tip opens the external orifice of the urethra. Further posteriorly and dorsally follows the hymen traversing the vaginal introitus. The bulbi vestibuli are located both sides to the vaginal introitus covered by the bulbo-cavernosi muscle (Fig. 2.5). The bulbo-cavernosi muscle therefore

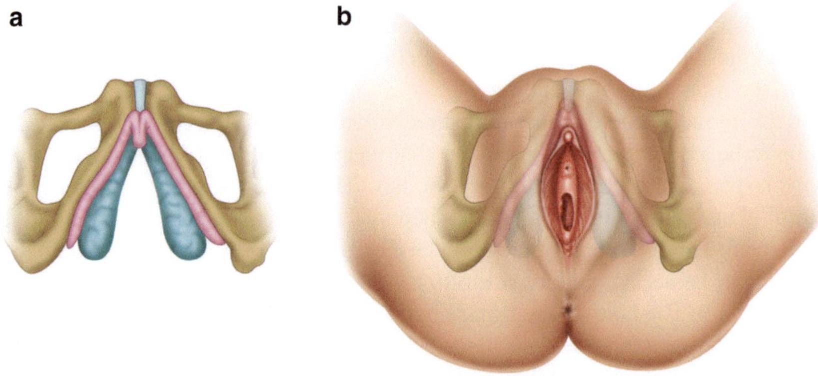

Fig. 2.5 Anatomic drawing of the clitoral organ (*colorations of original drawings from the author*). (**a**) (left) Drawing showing the clitoral organ flanked by the symphysis and the inferior rami of the pubic bone (description given from inside to outside): bulbi vestibuli being covered by the bulbo-cavernosi muscle; clitoris comprising the clitoral tip and clitoral bodies radially stretched by the suspensory ligament, as well as the clitoral crura paralleling the bulbi vestibuli at their lateral border. (**b**) (right) Illustration of clitoral topography projected on the vulva

surrounds the first third of the vagina and the urethra and merges both sides into the external sphincter muscle of the anus forming a figure of eight.

At the posterior-lateral vestibule, dorsally to the posterior part of the major labias, the Bartholin glands (major vestibular glands) are localized. Their excretory duct opens both sides at the posterior vestibule.

2.4.3 Region of the Genitofemoral Sulcus

The genitofemoral sulcus forms the border of the urogenital region against the thigh (Fig. 2.6a) and is of special significance for anatomic vulvar reconstruction [8]. Finally, it merges into the gluteal sulcus posteriorly and the inguinal sulcus anteriorly. At the transition zone, the gluteal sulcus sometimes splits into two arms.

Region of the genitofemoral-sulcus is unique in terms of vulvar reconstruction. It is of less subcutaneous fatty tissue providing thin and pliable skin with a stable vasculature and innervation. Due to these characteristics it is especially eligible for vulvar reconstruction compared to other regions, such as the medial thigh or the abdomen. Hair growth of that region, however, differs considerably and can be annoying when transposing this region into the vulva. Hair growth therefore should be addressed prior to surgery or secondarily depending on the postoperative accessibility.

Blood supply to the vulva is provided by mainly three vascular sources. These are from anterior to posterior: (1) the external pudendal arteries (Ae. pudendae externae) originating from the femoral artery (A. femoralis), (2) the obturator artery (A. obturatoria), and (3) the internal pudendal artery (A. pudenda interna), both of which originating from the internal iliac artery (A. iliaca interna).

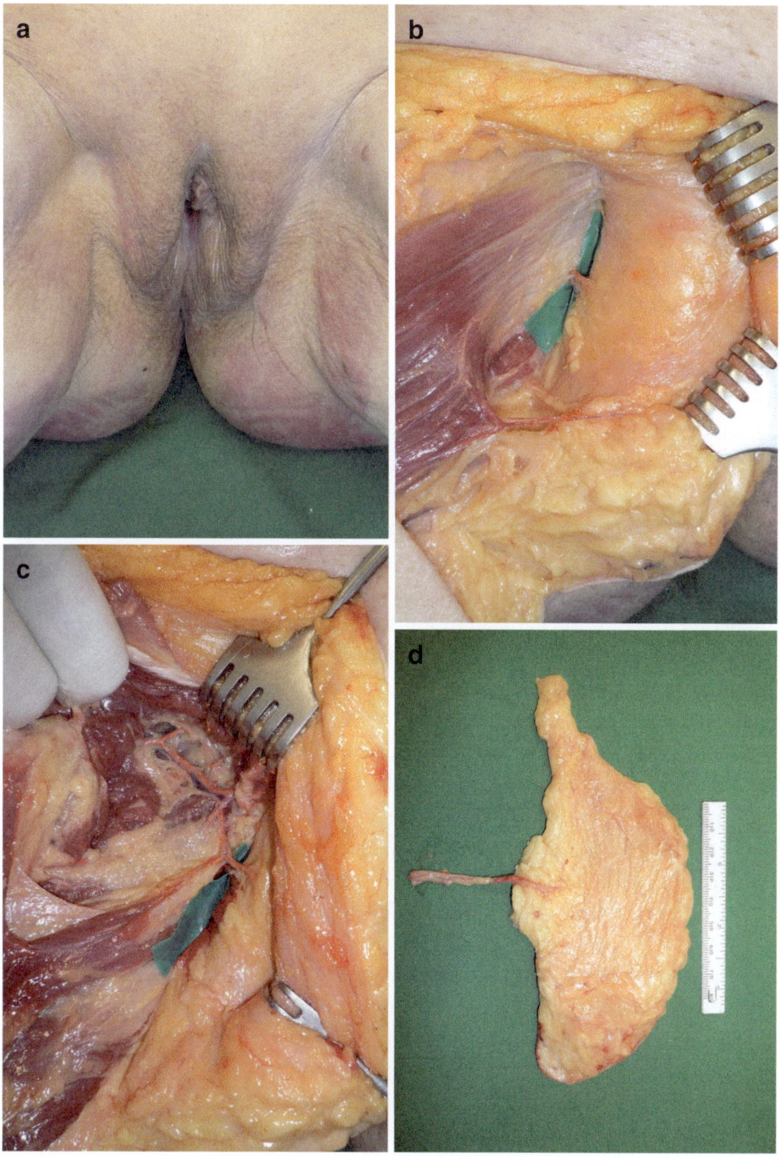

Fig. 2.6 Anatomic dissection detailing region of the genitofemoral sulcus. (**a**) (top left) View of the outer female genital prior to dissection; the genitofemoral sulcus forms a single line lateral to the major labias. (**b**) (top right) Subfascial dissection of the aOAP flap from anterolateral to posterior-medial under detection of the aOAP-perforator vessels (marked with a green background) piercing the aponeurosis of the gracilis muscle close to the inferior ramus of the pubic bone. (**c**) (bottom left) Further dissection of the aOAP-perforator vessels all the way down through musculature filling in the obturator foramen to its origin of the obturator artery and vein; course of the vessel is characterized by multiple side branches nourishing the musculature; note that arteries were filled beforehand with Pb3O4 (lead oxide) to ease dissection. (**d**) (bottom right) Isolated aOAP flap for descriptive purposes demonstrating extensions of the flap and potential length of the pedicle

When subdividing the pudendal region into thirds, the upper third is entered by extensions of the Ae. pudendae externae. The lower third is entered by the A. perinealis and the A. clitoridis, both of which originating from the A. pudenda interna. The A. clitoridis branches off the A. dorsalis clitoridis and the A. profunda clitoridis. The A. perinealis sends out the Rr. labiales posteriores.

The middle third is entered by a cutaneous branch originating from the R. anterior a. obturatoria, named the anterior obturator artery perforator (aOAP). The source vessel of the aOAP, the A. obturatoria, exits the pelvis as one out of four arteries originating from the A. iliaca interna. After passage of the obturator canal (canalis obturatorius) the obturator artery sends out the aOAP. Moreover, there is a distinctive anastomotic network formed by ramifications of the A. obturatoria and the A. circumflexa femoris medialis. The aOAP courses within the deep groin directed to the lateral border of the inferior pubic ramus while advancing to the skin of the sulcus genitofemoralis (Fig. 2.6b, c). Before reaching the skin, in 80% the vessel pierces the gracilis muscle proximally on the level of its thin aponeurosis as an indirect or musculocutaneous perforator 1.3 ± 0.3 cm near to the inferior pubic ramus. The vessel can be traced with a frequency of 20% passing the most proximal part of the gracilis muscle at its posterior border reflecting a direct course or septocutaneous perforator.

On its way to the skin the aOAP vessel traverses the fascia lata before entering the subcutaneous tissue of the genitofemoral sulcus. The vessel then branches while further advancing from medial to lateral. Length of the perforator measured down to its origin varied remarkably showing an average value of 5 ± 1.5 cm (Fig. 2.6c, d). Both septocutaneous and musculocutaneous anterior obturator perforators extend nearly perpendicularly to the subdermal plexus. Due to the vessel course, the aOAP flap can easily be made thinner, even though it is already the thinnest flap available right next to the vulva. With this in mind the deep layer of the subcutaneous tissue beyond the pedicle can be partly removed to further reduce the thickness of the flap and to allow for more flexibility. The subdermal or most superficial layer of the subcutaneous tissue embedding the extensions of the aOAP vessel, however, must be retained.

The aOAP flap forms the anatomic basis of a *perforator island flap* (Fig. 2.6d). It can be raised off the groin either epifascially or subfascially. Subfascial dissection, however, clearly facilitates elevation of the flap and allows for easy and safe identification of the aOAP vessel. The aOAP flap easily reaches defects of the vulva comprising the labia majora, the labia minora, the vestibule, the commissura labiorum anterior and posterior, and the fornix vaginae (vaginal introitus) pars anterior, pars posterior and partes lateralis on either the left or the right side, and last but not least the perineum.

2.5 Pathology

Tissue loss leads to anatomic alterations of form and function. Excision of the clitoral tip results in major damage to the sensory capacity of the female genital. That means that FGM/C type I already causes a catastrophic damage. Nobody will deny that fact, when realizing that excision of the male glans would have the same anatomic effect. Additional loss of the clitoral prepuce, minor labias, and major labias, of course, increases the damage and aggravates the deformity by major tissue loss restricting form and function. The damage culminates in FGM/C type III cases through disabling vulvovaginal function by narrowing the vestibule to a minimum. Any kind of FGM/C has a more or less devastating effect on the female genital showing overlapping and progressively amplifying pathologic effects.

Women suffering from FGM/C are severely burdened physically, socially, and emotionally. FGM/C patients frequently show neuromas of the stumps of the clitoral nerves flanking the remnants of the clitoral bodies [9]. Extended scarring, frequently including foreign bodies deriving from metal abrasion of inadequate cutting devices, or simply dirt particles, produces chronic inflammatory responses, pain, and discomfort. Moreover clitoral, epithelial, or retention cysts, and respective fistulas, are frequently found in region of the anterior vulva producing discomfort and inflammation.

A narrowed vestibule can lead to obstruction of the birth canal resulting in vulvoperineal rupture; genitourinary or genitorectal fistulas; disturbance of vaginal or urethral outflow; ascending infections of the vagina, the uterus, or the bladder; urgency; or dysuria. Prolonged obstructed delivery is not unusual in developing countries such as in Africa. As a result, extended tissue compression and subsequent vascular compromise may lead to multilayered tissue necrosis and fistulas. Furthermore, acquired fistulas may also result from the procedure itself, or consecutive infections, and may lead to continuous trickling of urine, fecal contamination of the vagina, genital odor, inflammation, and of course infection. Urine (ammonia) or fecal (digestive secretion or bacteria) leakages can significantly irritate the vagina, vulva, perineum, and surrounding skin sometimes leading to distinct dermatitis.

Tissue dynamics play an additional role and may get pathologic importance if anatomy is disturbed. The clitoral glans is usually fixed to the skin at the posterior border/opening of the clitoral prepuce and dynamically stretched and formed from within by the suspensory ligament [see 5, 6]. In case of amputation of the clitoral tip and part of the clitoral bodies in conjunction with the prepuce, tissue dynamics become unbalanced and the clitoral stump is consequently retracted to the pubic bone by the suspensory ligament. This intrinsic maneuver is typically seen in all FGM/C types involving the clitoris; these are FGM/C type I to III and potentially type IV.

Literature

1. Hafferl A. Lehrbuch der topographischen Anatomie. Berlin: Springer; 1957. p. 1–891.
2. Di Marino V, Lepidi H. Anatomic study of the clitoris and the bulbo-clitoral organ. Heidelberg: Springer; 2014. p. 1–152.
3. O'Connell HE, Sanjeevan KV, Hutson J. Anatomy of the clitoris. J Urol. 2005;174:1189–95.
4. Puppo V. Anatomy and physiology of the clitoris, vestibular bulbs, and labia minora with a review of the female orgasm and the prevention of female sexual dysfunction. Clin Anat. 2013;26:134–52.

5. Temesvary N. Die regio clitoridis. Arch Gynakol. 1924;122:102–28.
6. Rees MA, O'Connel HE, Plenter RJ, Hutson JM. The suspensory ligament of the clitoris: connective tissue supports of the erectile tissue of the female urogenital region. Clin Anat. 2000;13:397–403.
7. Lax H. Stoeckels Lehrbuch der Gynäkologie. Leipzig: S Herzel Verlag; 1967. p. 1–33.
8. O'Dey DM, Bozkurt A, Pallua N. The anterior Obturator Artery Perforator (aOAP) flap: surgical anatomy and application of a method for vulvar reconstruction. Gynecol Oncol. 2010;119:526–30. Epub 2010 Sep 24.
9. Abdulcadir J, Tille JC, Petignat P. Management of painful clitoral neuroma after female genital mutilation/cutting. Reprod Health. 2017;14:22. https://doi.org/10.1186/s12978-017-0288-3.

Procedures

3

3.1 General Perspective

Inspiration is progress, and progress is inspiration. Reconstructive procedures must be inspiring for both the patient and the surgeon. Once perceived, the spirit of reconstructive surgery will be present likewise initiating intrinsic motivation for an overall perfect result with respect to form and function.

Procedures invented by the author that are presented in this book enable to rebuild important anatomic features of the outer female genital. They thereby provide significant improvements in line with physical restoration, and also lead to a potential support of psychological stability of the patients. Procedures under focus are complex, might be not easily performed, and are also regarded as time consuming. Efforts and time however are relative weighted factors as the result is outstanding. The surgeon needs to be focused on both anatomy and the cutting edge of techniques to bring out the best result possible. It is therefore all about medical attitude, in a certain sense, to gain the best result for our patients promising their entire recovery.

3.1.1 Surgical Instruments

Vulvar and clitoral reconstruction should be performed using fine plastic surgical instruments and supporting equipment. These include a magnifying loop 4.0× or higher, good lightning, fine and blunt retractors, as well as sharp one- and

Electronic Supplementary Material The online version of this chapter (doi:10.1007/978-3-030-02168-9_3) contains supplementary material, which is available to authorized users.

D. m. O´Dey, *Vulvar Reconstruction Following Female Genital Mutilation/Cutting (FGM/C) and other Acquired Deformities*,
https://doi.org/10.1007/978-3-030-02168-9_3

two-prong retractors, and furthermore blunt dissection instruments like small curved over-holds, nontraumatic and fine sharp forceps, fine sharp scissors, and of course micro-instruments.

3.1.2 Planning

The complexity of the procedure must be considered prior to surgery. Planning on the patient by means of markings is imperative. It is important to go mentally through all steps of the procedure in the particular patient tailored to her individual anatomic preconditions. Then it will be possible to find solutions before anticipated problems arise during surgery. This will clearly contribute to efficiency of the procedure.

3.1.3 Anesthesia and Preparation

Reconstruction of the vulva and the clitoris is best accomplished under general or regional anesthesia. Additional infiltration of local anesthetics, such as Xylonest with Adrenalin 1:200,000, eases preparation, clears the operative field, and supports pain reduction. Prophylactic antibiotics and vulvar shaving should be standardly performed. Bladder catheterization could be hindering intraoperatively and should therefore be done at the end of the procedure or temporarily during the procedure.

3.1.4 Positioning

The patient is placed in the lithotomy position and marked on the skin according to the regular vascular anatomy (Fig. 3.1a). Detection with a Doppler probe and marking of the perforator vessel to be safely included in the skin island of the aOAP flap are of vital importance to the survival of the tissue. Lateral pressure of the stirrups against the head of the fibula should be avoided to prevent pressure against the peroneal nerve. Patient's buttocks are pulled inferiorly down to the border of the operating table to provide both an optimal view and access. The surgeon must take great care that the patient's legs are sufficiently padded and positioned. Due to the duration of the procedure I strongly recommend to temporarily interrupt the procedure and subsequently change position of the legs temporarily just to prevent vascular or pressure-dependent complications of the legs. In addition, standard *intermittent pneumatic compression* (IPC) garment extending from knee to ankle is recommended both sided as well as pre- and postoperative anticoagulants. The surgeon should be placed in a comfortable position sitting upright in front of the patient (Fig. 3.1b) supported by an assistant standing cranial to the legs sideways on the left or the right side (Fig. 3.2).

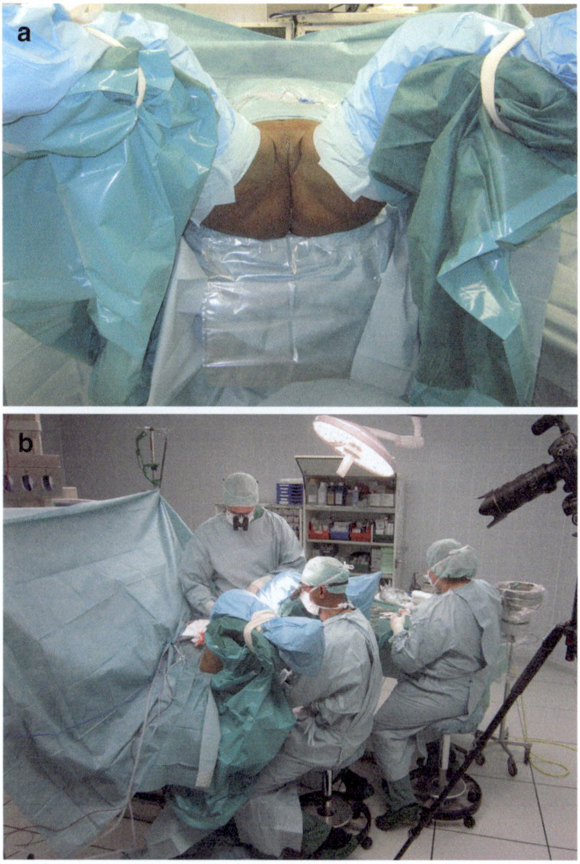

Fig. 3.1 Operative setting I. (**a**) (top) Sterile setting and placement of the patient in the lithotomy position; angled legs should be ready to be changed in position during operation to prevent for nerval and/or vascular damage of the lower legs; for this purpose additional intermittent pneumatic compression (IPC) therapy should be beneficial. (**b**) (bottom) Surgeon should be placed in a comfortable position sitting upright in front of the patient

3.1.5 Perforator Dissection

Perforator dissection requires patience (Fig. 2.6c), confident dissection skills, gentle tissue handling, greatest attention to hemostasis to guaranty for a bloodless operative field, and the ability to have everything in sight. The aOAP vessel is vulnerable and it can be easily damaged by dissection, especially when opening the firm aponeurosis of the gracilis muscle (Fig. 2.6b) or moving forward beyond the aponeurosis. Before consequently cutting the fascia to further work out the pedicle, subaponeurotic course of the aOAP vessel should be anticipated visually by gently spreading the aponeurotic slit. Then the pedicle can be safely freed from the aponeurosis and be further dissected down to its origin (Fig. 2.6c). Vessel clips best perform the control of side branches. Smaller vessels and capillaries are controlled with bipolar coagulation. Retracting encountered side branches or connective tissue bands usually cause resistance around the pedicle or tension at the pedicle during

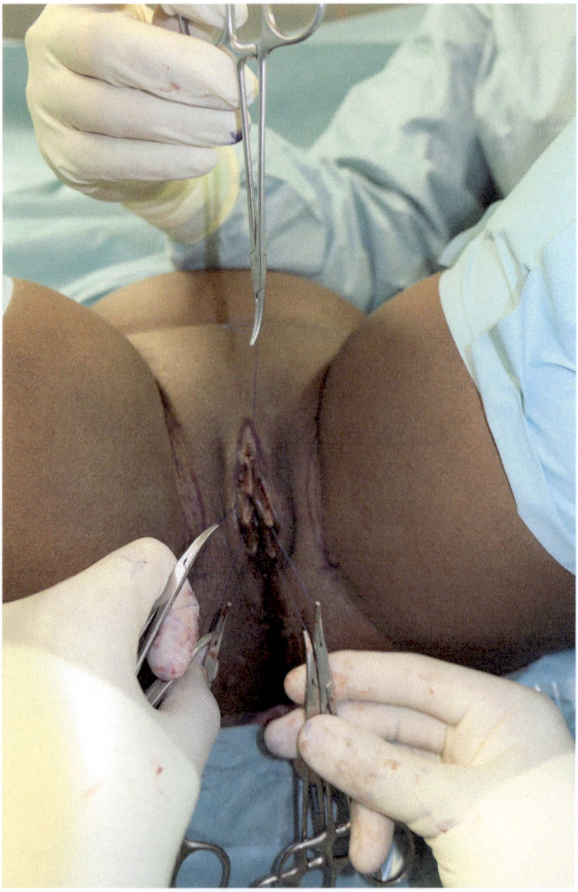

Fig. 3.2 Operative setting II. Positioning of the assistant standing sideways and cranial to the legs of the patient; enabling the surgeon for unimpaired handling within the operation field; note that it is strictly forbidden to rest arms on legs of the patient to prevent nerve impairment

dissection. The pedicle must be freed from these restrictions to gain mobility. Irrigating the pedicle with papaverine at the end of the dissection solves reactive vasospasm.

3.2 Clitoral Reconstruction

Clitoral reconstruction takes a key part in vulvar reconstruction due to the functional completion of the outer female genital and its lasting importance for bodily integrity. The clitoral organ reflects a unique sensory capacity for the female organism based on an interacting network of the peripheral and central nervous system. Due to the fact that the clitoral tip transfers the external stimulus over fine endings of the dorsal clitoral nerves to the central nervous system, fine microsurgical reconstruction of the clitoral tip is clearly recommended in case of ablative procedures such as FGM/C. As in peripheral nerve surgery the best result should then be expected from tension-free and directed nerve sprouting covered by healthy tissue preventing undirected regeneration. Besides functional reconstruction form is essential as it usually supports function. The following techniques do respect both form and function of the reconstructed clitoral organ through the Omega-Domed flap and the NMCS procedure (neurotizing and molding of the clitoral stump).

3.2.1 General Perspective

The clitoral region is a complex area presenting several anatomic details, all of which should be addressed by reconstructive procedures [1, 2]. With respect to this claim an anatomical normal clitoral region should comprise an identifiable prepuce, a coronal clitoral sulcus with flanking skin folds, and a reinnervated clitoral glans. The clitoral glans should further be fine rather than bulky and should show and keep an identifiable projection (Fig. 3.3a–f). From a reconstructive point of view form of the clitoral tip does matter. Due to dynamics of the tissue projection of the reconstructed clitoral tip decreases slightly with time. That's why a little overcorrection of clitoral tip projection is almost always advisable. Anatomic reconstruction, however, is time consuming. Less concern about anatomic form and function may therefore also be reasonable [3–5] but generally worth aspiring to.

3.2.2 Reconstruction of the Prepuce Using the Omega-Domed Flap (OD Flap)

The need for surgical repair of anatomic subunits of the clitoral region depends on the complexity of tissue loss. The female prepuce has several important functions and is a significant anatomic detail to be considered reconstructively. Concerning FGM/C type I to III, the prepuce is almost always involved. In contrast to other techniques rejecting a buttonhole-like skin region to get surgical access to the remaining clitoral organ overlying the clitoral stump [see 5, 6], it can conceptually be used instead to gain access as well as to form a new clitoral prepuce.

3.2.2.1 Importance of the Clitoral Prepuce and the OD Flap

Attempts to reconstruct the clitoral prepuce should address mechanical protection and conceptual aesthetics of the newly formed clitoral tip. It should therefore complete the surgical objectives of anatomic reconstruction and likewise increases the functional and aesthetic benefits for FGM/C patients (Fig. 3.4).

For functional protective and aesthetic purposes I invented a local flap technique called the Omega-Domed flap (OD flap) for prepuce reconstruction. The contour of the flap conceptually forms an "omega" following anterior transposition and then creates a "dome" over the clitoral stump when it is folded on itself (Figs. 3.4 and 3.6). These characteristics were decisive for naming of the "Omega-Domed flap

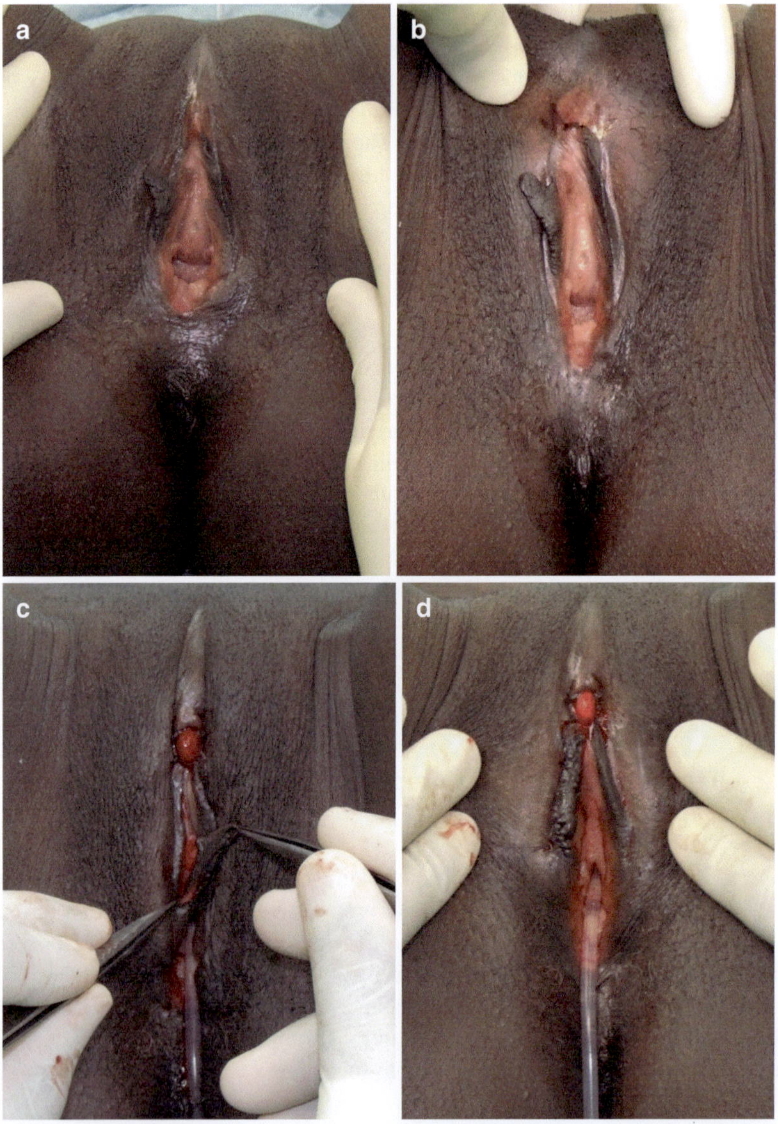

Fig. 3.3 Clitoral reconstruction in a FGM/C type II 50-year-old woman. (**a**) (top left) Preoperative view showing the FGM/C type II amputated upper third of the vulva; additionally the right minor labia was detached halfway anteriorly. (**b**) (top right) Preoperative view showing the marking of the OD flap in the region of the new position of the clitoral tip. (**c**) (middle left) Intraoperative view after microsurgical reconstruction of the clitoral tip with the NMCS procedure, prepuce reconstruction with the OD flap; minor labial repair on the right side by transpositioning and grafting of the loose anterior part to both its basis and its root is shown. (**d**) (middle right) Intraoperative view after microsurgical reconstruction of the clitoral tip with the NMCS procedure, prepuce reconstruction with the OD flap, and completed reconstruction of the right minor labia. (**e**) (bottom left) Postoperative view under slight tension 1 year after reconstruction showing a stable and still normalized anatomy with a fine projection of the clitoral tip, and natural contour of the prepuce and minor labias. (**f**) (bottom right) Same patient at rest 1 year after reconstruction; note the overall normal and appealing impression of the vulvar contour

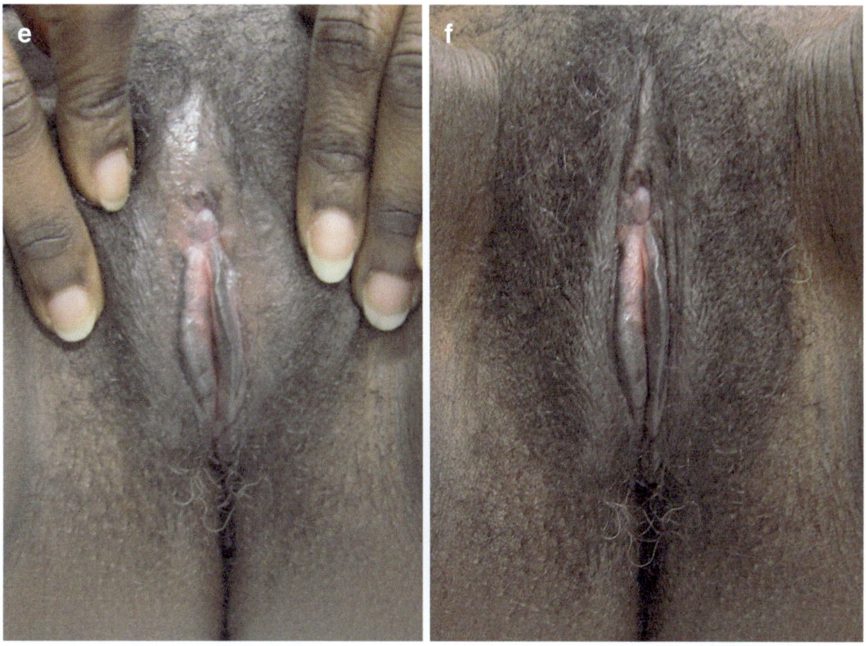

Fig. 3.3 (continued)

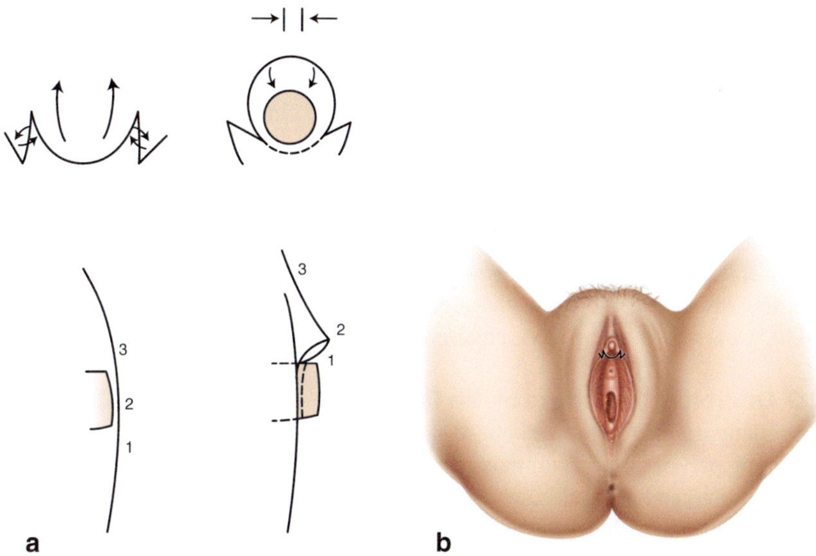

Fig. 3.4 Schematic drawings of the Omega-Domed flap (*colorations of original drawings from the author*). (**a**) (left) The OD flap is a composition of an opposing Z-plasty flanking a central semicircular transposition flap. The transposed limbs of the opposing Z-plasty and elevated central transposition flap give way to the clitoral stump (crosshatched circle). The central semicircular transposition flap is domed over the reconstructed clitoral tip (crosshatched area). (**b**) (right) Illustration of the incisional pattern of the OD flap projected on the vulva

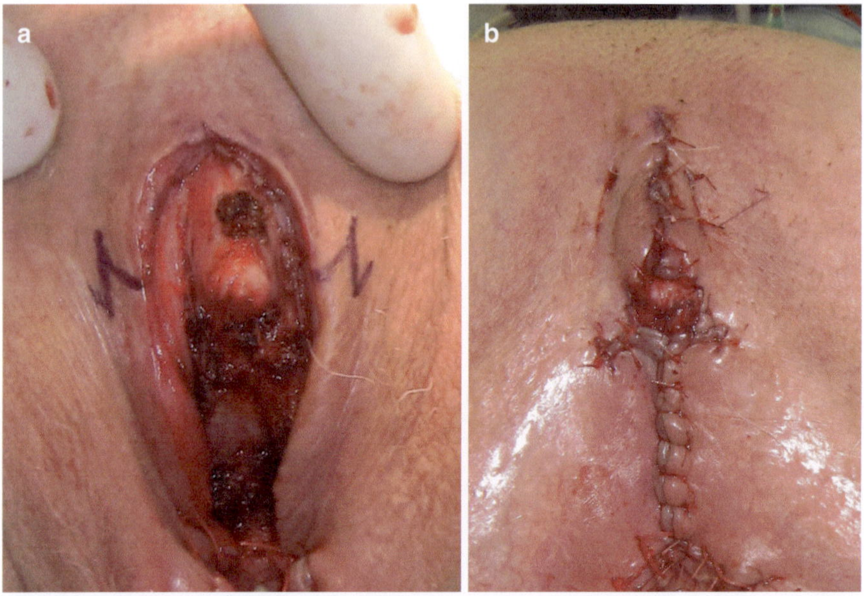

Fig. 3.5 63-Year-old woman with carcinoma of the clitoral region. (**a**) (left) Intraoperative view after excision of the carcinoma and marking of the OD flap split into halves. (**b**) (right) Reconstruction of the prepuce with the both sides split OD flap showing the centered fine clitoral tip

(OD flap)." For FGM/C type III patients I tailored the OD flap concept adjusted to the aOAP flaps. In those FGM/C type III patients this modified OD flap technique can be used to similarly restore anatomy of the prepuce as in type I and II patients using the scarred skin anterior-ventrally overlying the clitoral stump. The anterior-medial-most parts of the aOAP flaps instead are then applied for this purpose (Fig. 3.5). Geometrically the standard OD flap is virtually split into halves allocated on both sides of the aOAP flaps. For descriptive purposes I call this maneuver the "split-OD flap technique." It requires, however, in-depth understanding and experience with the aOAP flap procedure with special regard to vasculature. In consequence, the subdermal plexus in the region of the aOAP-flap-splitting procedure should be preserved to rule out vascular complications.

3.2.2.2 Operative Procedure of the OD Flap

With the patient generally anesthetized and placed in the lithotomy position, the anterior-most part of clitoral stump is palpated and recognized. Then the OD flap is planned and marked on the skin where the new clitoral tip should be best anatomically located (Fig. 3.6), that is, the medial to inferior third of the symphysis. Planning of the OD flap must then consider general rules of vascularity important for randomized local skin flaps. For this purpose the transverse diameter of the central transposition flap is set between 15 and 20 mm. The limbs of the Z-plasties should be nearly half the diameter of the central transposition flap. This central part forms a semicircular, anteriorly based transposition flap (Fig. 3.4), flanked by a bilateral

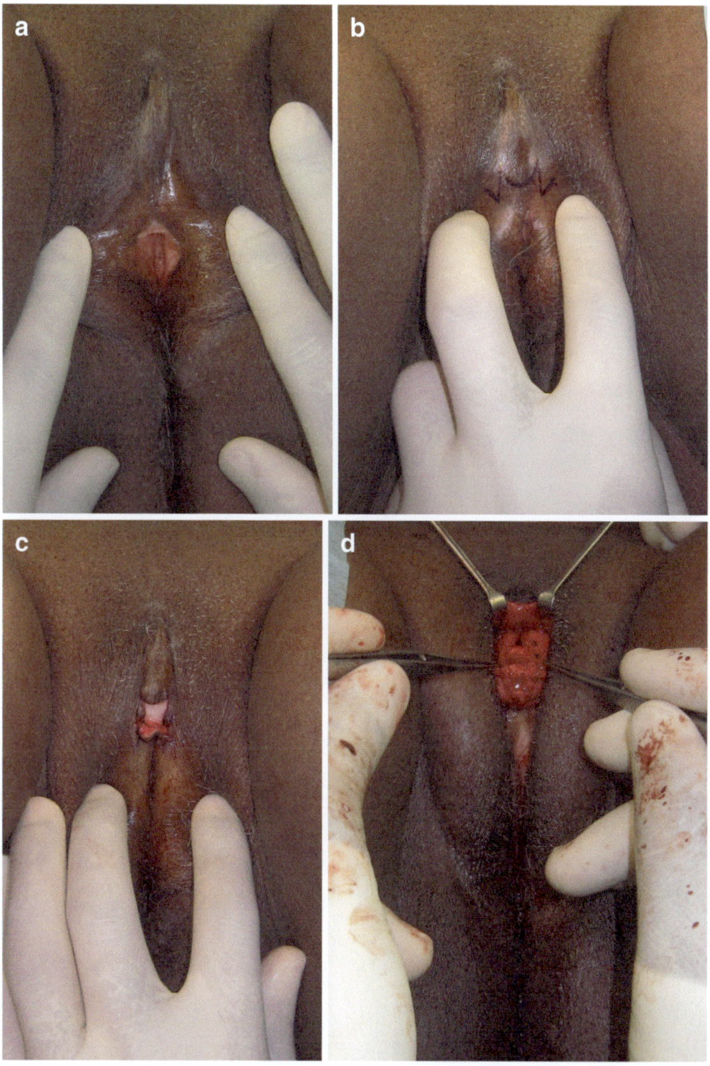

Fig. 3.6 55-Year-old patient with clitoral and prepuce reconstruction after FGM/C type II; the OD flap and the NMCS procedure are shown. (**a**) (rooftop left) Preoperative view showing absence of the clitoral tip, prepuce, and minor labias. (**b**) (rooftop right) Preoperative view showing marking of the OD flap on the skin. (**c**) (top left) Intraoperative view after incision and elevation of the OD flap demonstrating the stump of the clitoris surrounded by fibrous tissue/scar. (**d**) (top right) Intraoperative view showing the stump of the clitoris after excision of the clitoral scarring and mobilization of the clitoral bodies; forceps grasp the clitoral nerves prior to NMCS procedure. (**e**) (middle left) Intraoperative view after NMCS procedure showing the formed clitoral tip and closed bed of the formerly retracted clitoral stump. (**f**) (middle right) Intraoperative view demonstrating the interdermal sutures to form the wall of the anteriorly fading prepuce; note that the nonabsorbable braided sutures are placed interdermally covered by the skin. (**g**) (bottom left) Final result intraoperatively at rest; note the fine clitoral tip, and the clitoral wall fading anteriorly. (**h**) (bottom right) Final result intraoperatively with slight spreading of the vestibule; note the clitoral wall domed over the newly formed clitoral tip with the OD flap. (**i**) (basement left) Follow-up after 3 weeks postoperatively; note that re-epithelialization of the clitoral tip is almost done still showing a reddish aspect

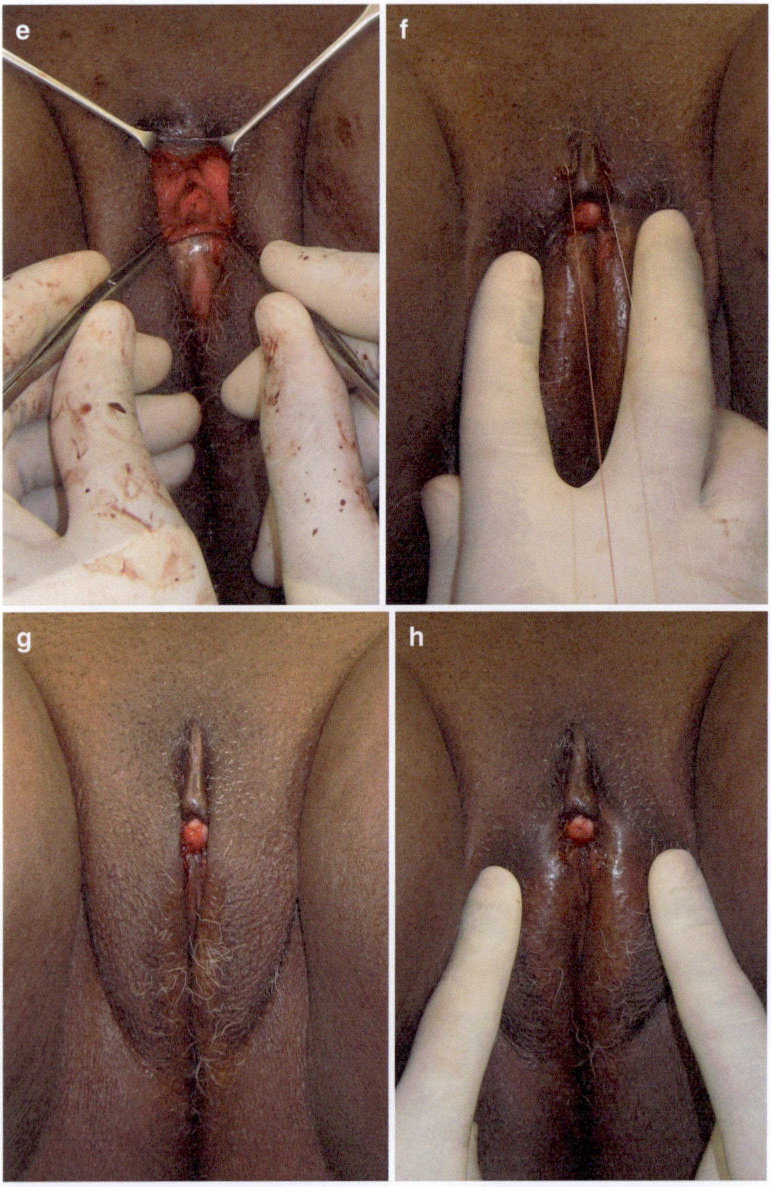

Fig. 3.6 (continued)

Fig. 3.6 (continued)

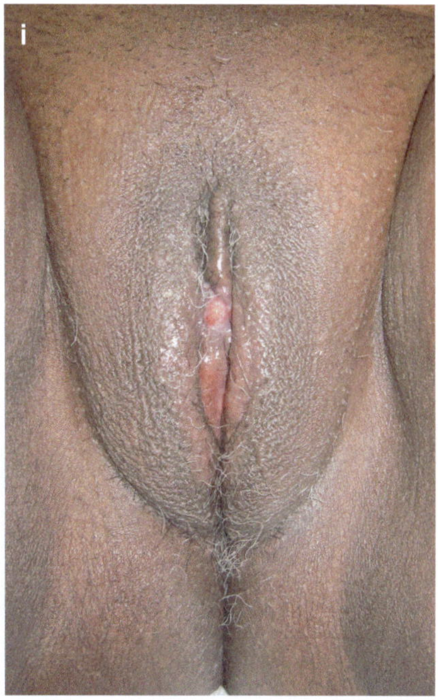

Z-plasty (Figs. 3.4 and 3.6). So, both Z-plasties are related to each other medially. The Z-plasties within the OD flap allow for lifting the central transposition flap anteriorly while narrowing the harvest side.

Local anesthetic with vasoconstrictors (1:400,000) is infiltrated after flap planning is completed. Incision is performed along the planned cutaneous incision line and deepened into the subcutaneous tissue (Fig. 3.6). All parts of the flap are then carefully elevated subcutaneously beginning with the central part. Care is taken for safe vasculature of the subdermal plexus and individual branches found in that region. The flap is carefully elevated to its base.

After having completed flap elevation, the clitoral stump usually represented by remnants of the clitoral bodies (see NMCS Procedure Sect. 3.2.3) is then explored and freed from fibrotic tissue and scars (Fig. 3.6c, d). Superficial and deep parts of the suspensory ligament retaining the clitoral stump are completely cut all the way down to the symphysic bone at the anterior-most part of the retracted stump. This maneuver is necessary to gain mobility of the tissue (Fig. 3.6d). The clitoral stump then is dissected out of the surrounding tissue likewise isolating the remaining clitoral bodies and accompanying dorsal clitoral nerves and vessels.

Finally, the central part of the OD flap is folded on itself (Fig. 3.4), sutured to the upper edge of the newly formed clitoral tip being reconstructed beforehand with the NMCS procedure (see Sect. 3.2.3), and thereby domed over it (Figs. 3.4 and 3.6e, f). The clitoral tip then is kept uncovered at its ventral surface of course, to allow for healing by secondary intention likewise offering the most possible sensory capacity of it. Placing interdermal 4.0 or 5.0 braided nonabsorbable mattress sutures resembles the tapered anterior part of the clitoral prepuce (Fig. 3.6f). Care must be taken,

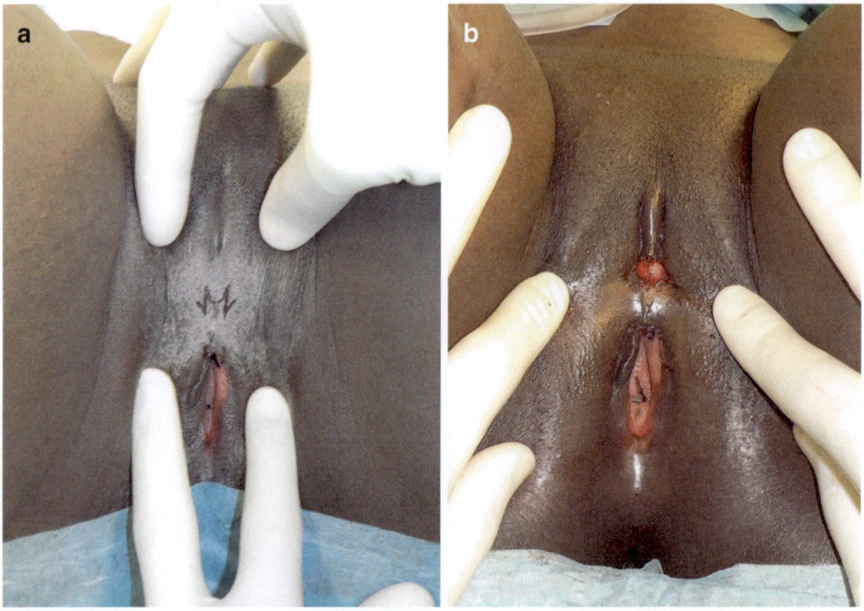

Fig. 3.7 23-Year-old patient with FGM/C type II. (**a**) (left) Preoperative view showing marking of the OD flap anteriorly and that of a opposed Z-plasty at the anterior border of the vestibule. (**b**) (right) Intraoperative view after reconstruction of the clitoral region with the OD flap, NMCS procedure, and release of tension at the anterior vestibule with the opposed Z-plasty

however, to avoid immoderate tightness of the interdermal sutures to create a natural appearance of the newly formed lateral walls of the prepuce (Fig. 3.6). Depending on the scar characteristics found, it is sometimes beneficial to place a double-Z-plasty or dancing-man plasty as an occasional part of the procedure, posterior to the OD flap (Fig. 3.7), to reduce tension at the anterior vestibule.

All in all the OD flap technique clearly contributes to create natural conditions of the clitoral region while supporting function of the microsurgically reconstructed clitoral tip. It is therefore very appropriate for FGM/C type I to III patients and of course shows further indications for patients presenting with other deformities of the outer female genital.

3.2.3 Reconstruction of the Clitoral Glans: The Neurotizing and Molding of the Clitoral Stump (NMCS) Procedure (Video 3.1)

The clitoral glans is comparable with a fingertip as a region of complex sensitivity built up by fine-sprouted endings of two main nerves—called the dorsal clitoral nerves. Reinnervation of a new clitoral glans formed out of the clitoral corpora following excisions such as in FGM/C procedures requires best tissue conditions. From a microsurgical point of view that means providing unimpaired tension-free nerve edges covered by healthy tissue able to sprout out directionally into a conical shaped tip.

In FGM/C patients involving the clitoris, excision of neuromas and scars off the clitoral stump should be performed sharply delivering precise and smooth cuts (Fig. 3.8). This usually leaves the shortened nerve ends in their anatomic position several millimeters apart from each other (Fig. 3.8c, d). Further dissection of the clitoral stump on the level of the clitoral bodies needs meticulous care taken to safeguard these nerves flanking the clitoral bodies superficially at the 11 and 13 o'clock positions (Fig. 3.9). Dissection of the nerves posteriorly is therefore performed microsurgically over a distance of around 10–15 mm on both sides using fine spring-style microscissors and forceps to gain structural mobility for later tension-free transposition of the nerves into the newly formed clitoral tip (Fig. 3.9d).

After dissection of the clitoral nerves has been successfully completed, diagonal tunnels are created bluntly over several millimeters with fine-tip scissors on both sides starting bilaterally at the middle surface of the cut edge of the clitoral bodies directed toward the 11 and 13 o'clock positions. The dorsal clitoral nerves are then

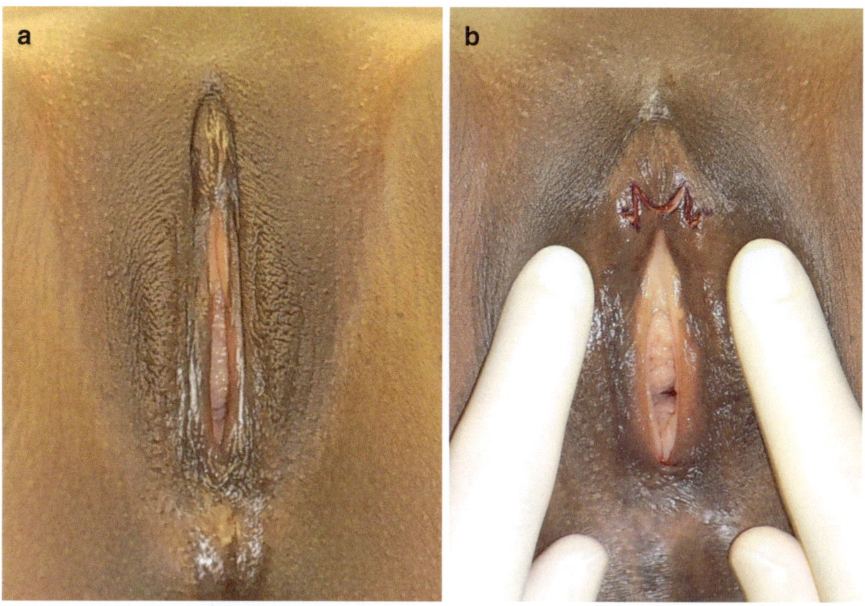

Fig. 3.8 30-Year-old patient with FGM/C type II. (**a**) (top left) View of the outer female genital prior to reconstruction; the clitoral prepuce, clitoral tip, and minor labias are absent. (**b**) (top right) Intraoperative view after marking and incision of the OD flap anterior to the vestibule. (**c**) (middle left) Clear cut of the clitoral stump directed to the symphysis on the level of the clitoral bodies by using sharp scissors. (**d**) (middle right) Microsurgical repair of the clitoral tip by using the NMCS procedure; note that the suture material is a nonabsorbable monofilament 9.0/10.0 microsuture. (**e**) (bottom left) Intraoperative view after complete reconstruction, showing a fine and adequate projected clitoral tip as well as naturally formed prepuce. (**f**) (bottom right) Follow-up examination 1 year after reconstruction still demonstrating a good projection of the completely re-epithelized clitoral tip (brownish as the surrounding skin)

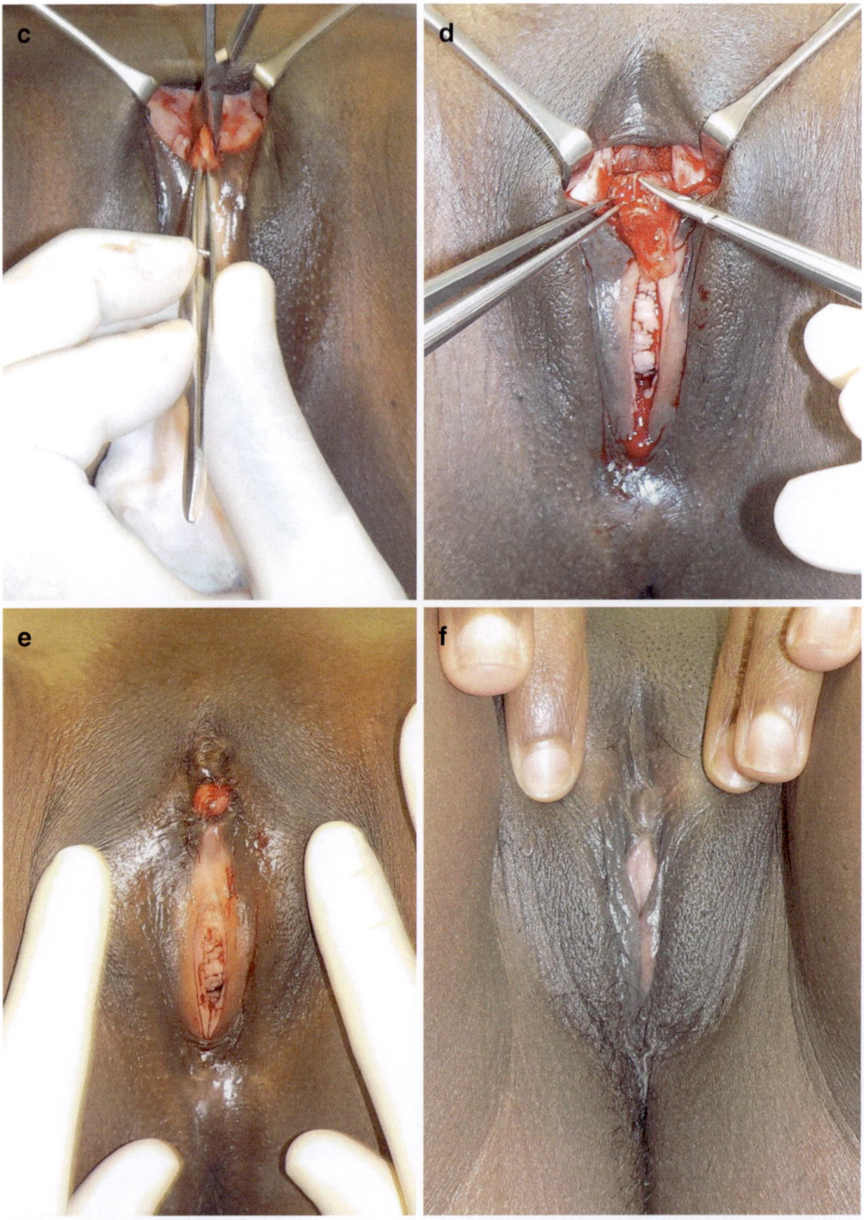

Fig. 3.8 (continued)

passed through the tunnels tension free bringing them from outside to inside entering the middle surface of the clitoral bodies on both sides (Fig. 3.9e). The nerves are then fixed epineurally to the gate using 9.0 or 10.0 microsutures to prevent them from sliding backwards. The tunica albuginea is then used to cover the neurotized area while creating a conical shaped tip.

This neurotizing maneuver allows for sprouting of the nerves into the newly formed clitoral tip surrounded by well-vascularized tissue rather than fading blindly at the outer surface of the clitoral bodies. The clitoral stump represented by the clitoral bodies must, however, show clear-cut edges without scarring to offer the best conditions for nerve ingrowth.

Alternatively the freed nerves can be transposed also tension free directly over the side depending on the topographic relations. After passing the nerves onto the central surface of the clitoral bodies they are fixed microsurgically using 9.0 or 10.0 single-knot microsutures (Fig. 3.9e, f). Then the envelope of the clitoral bodies

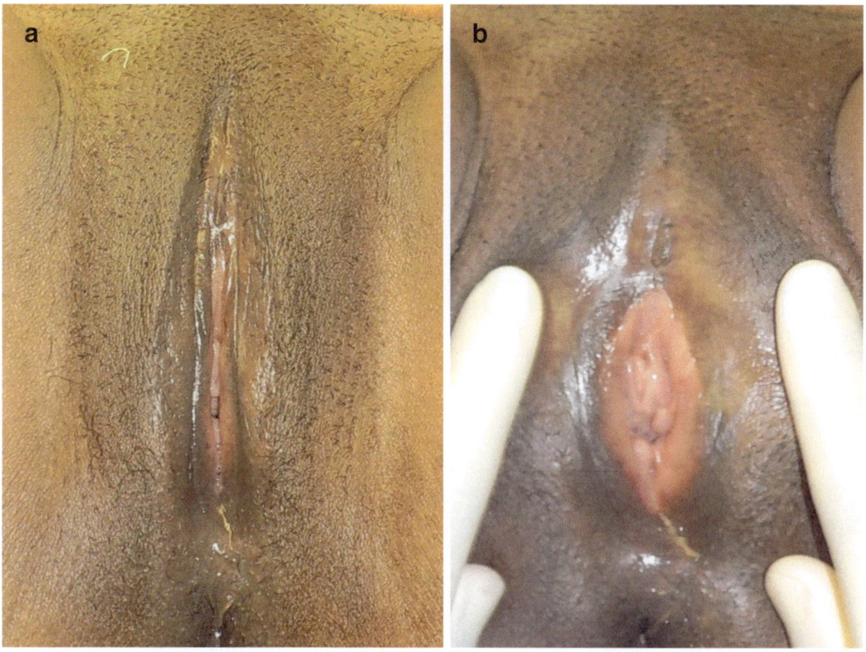

Fig. 3.9 30-Year-old patient with clitoris and prepuce reconstruction after FGM/C type II; the OD flap and the NMCS procedure are shown. (**a**) (rooftop left) Preoperative view at rest showing absence of the clitoral tip, prepuce, and minor labias. (**b**) (rooftop right) Preoperative view under slight tension. (**c**) (top left) Intraoperative view after incision and elevation of the OD flap; the released stump of the clitoris on the level of the clitoral bodies cleared of any scar is demonstrated. (**d**) (top right) Intraoperative view showing the formerly retracted stump of the clitoris after excision of fibrous tissue and mobilization of the clitoral bodies; forceps grasping the mobilized clitoral nerves for the NMCS procedure. (**e**) (middle left) Intraoperative view during the NMCS procedure showing the dissected tunnels formed for pull through of the clitoral nerves. (**f**) (middle right) Intraoperative view demonstrating the microsurgical integration of the clitoral nerves into the center of the clitoral bodies. (**g**) (bottom left) Intraoperative view demonstrating adaptation of the clitoral cone harboring the reinserted clitoral nerves. (**h**) (bottom right) Final result intraoperatively under slight spreading of the vestibule; note the fine diameter of the clitoral tip. (**i**) (basement left) Final result intraoperatively at rest; note the fine diameter of the clitoral tip and the overall natural characteristic of the clitoral region

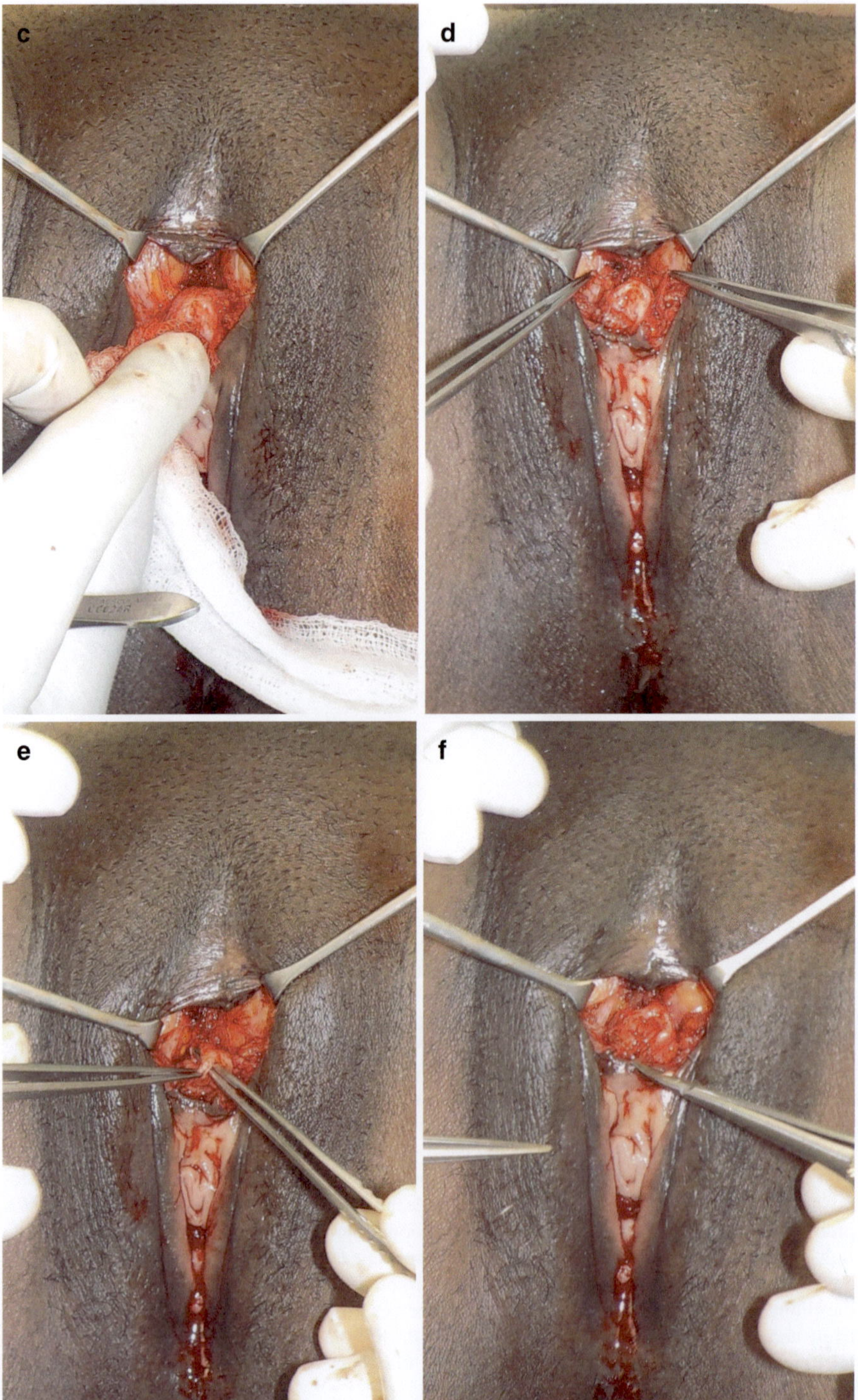

Fig. 3.9 (continued)

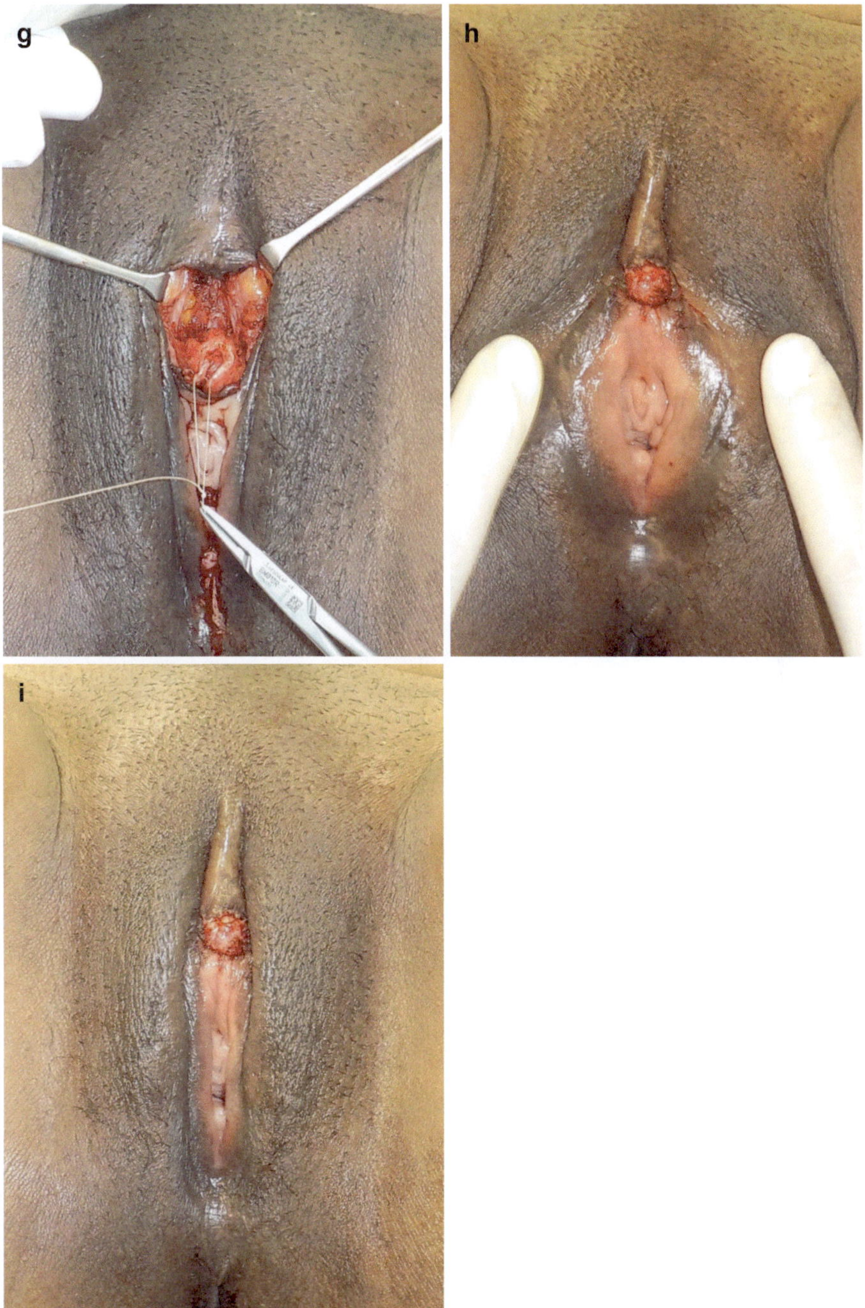

Fig. 3.9 (continued)

formed by the tunica albuginea is used to create a cone-shaped tip (Fig. 3.9g) using braided and resorbable 6.0 or 7.0 sutures. This will then enable for centripetal nerve sprouting out of the dorsal clitoral nerves likewise neurotizing the newly formed clitoral tip from within.

In total, I call the described surgical procedure the "NMCS procedure" meaning "neurotizing and molding of the clitoral stump" (Fig. 3.10).

The newly formed and microsurgically reconstructed clitoral tip is then transposed ventrally and anchored to its new position in between the opposite Z-plasties of the OD flap. Anchoring is performed with deep resorbable inverted 5.0 monofilament sutures followed by superficially placed resorbable 6.0 braided sutures.

As described in Sect. 3.2.2 the central transposition flap of the OD flap is then domed over the clitoral tip by using resorbable braided 5.0 single-knot sutures. The procedure is finalized by forming of the preputial wall (Figs. 3.6f and 3.10d). Forming the preputial wall can be accomplished by placing carefully tightened

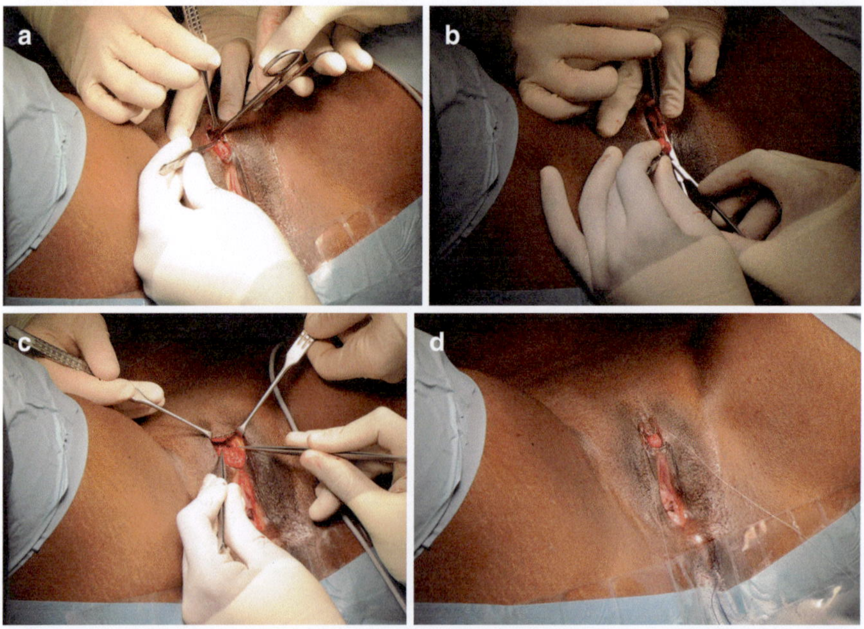

Fig. 3.10 Reconstruction of the clitoral region using the OD flap and the NMCS procedure in a 30-year-old woman with FGM/C type II. (**a**) (top left) Intraoperative view showing dissection of the clitoral stump by cutting the suspensory ligament to the symphysis. (**b**) (top right) Intraoperative view demonstrating a clear cut to the clitoral stump providing a well-defined surface of both the clitoral bodies and the clitoral nerves. (**c**) (bottom left) Dissection of the clitoral nerve grasps with fine forceps. (**d**) (bottom right) Result after NMCS procedure and creation of a cone-shaped clitoral tip; note the prepared interdermal suture to form the wall of the prepuce

interdermal sutures anterior to the OD flap (Fig. 3.11). For this maneuver I prefer braided nonabsorbable 4.0 mattress sutures. The sutures are positioned after placing stab incisions opposed to each other. A maximum of two sutures should be sufficient for this purpose.

Improvement of clitoral perception is of main interest concerning clitoral reconstruction. Reinnervation, however, is a matter of time and needs patience on both sides of the patient and the surgeon. To evaluate the progress of reinnervation of the clitoral tip, I used to ask my patients periodically while palpating the tip about the subjective alteration of clitoral perception obtained through the NMCS procedure while comparing it with their sensitivity before reconstruction. Due to the fact that descriptive ranking of clitoral perception is difficult in detail, I try to simplify assessment by providing an abstraction scale as shown in Fig. 3.12. Functional outcome after clitoral reconstruction can be objectified thereby through a quantitative enquiry. The scale used ranges from "0" corresponding to a sad smiley, meaning no perception as frequently found preoperatively, up to "10" represented by a happy smiley, meaning a maximum of perception. I always ask them to remember their starting point before reconstruction first, and then to compare it with their actual impression of gained clitoral perception. It is remarkable that almost all patients assure that they would rank their gained clitoral perception with an "8." A few declare a "10" or even a "12" just to underline that they are overwhelmed by their clitoral feeling. These moments, of course, are great. I'm convinced that this remarkable outcome observed following the NMCS procedure is closely linked to the microsurgical approach optimizing direct nerve ingrowth in the midst of the newly formed clitoral tip.

3.3 Complex Vulvar Reconstruction Following FGM Type III (Infibulation)

3.3.1 General Perspective

From a reconstructive point of view the main problem with FGM type III is cross-functional tissue loss resembling both partial vulvectomy and clitorectomy. Reconstruction therefore should address different anatomic needs. Concerning anatomy there should be three key features to be addressed when attending to structurally normalize the vulva. The first out of these three key features is the need of elasticity reestablished by soft, thin, and pliable tissue added to the vulvar vestibule resembling the transition zone of the major and the minor labias. The second is functional reconstruction of a fine cone-shaped

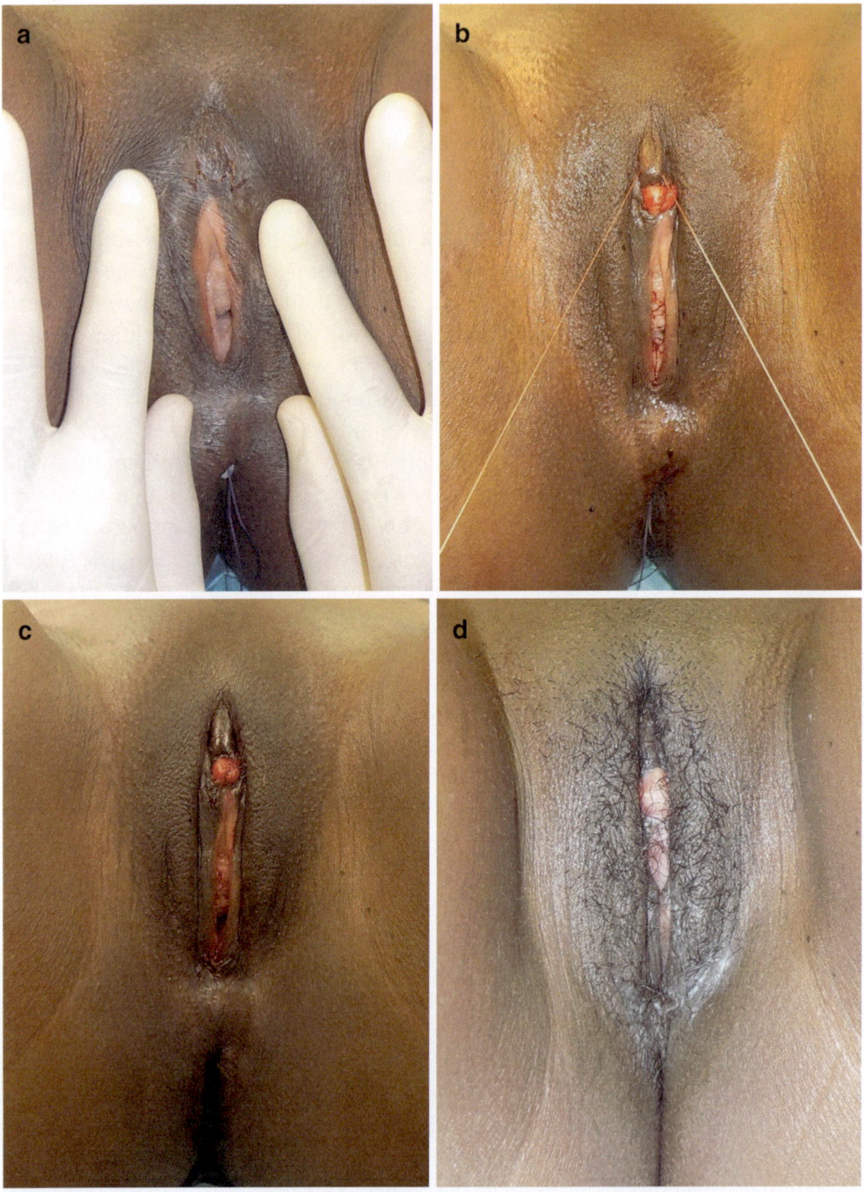

Fig. 3.11 Reconstruction of the clitoral region in a 30-year-old woman with FGM/C type II. (**a**) (top left) Preoperative view showing the absence of the prepuce, and clitoral tip; Drawing of the OD flap has already been done. (**b**) (top right) Intraoperative view after reconstruction of the clitoral tip with the NMCS procedure. (**c**) (bottom left) Postoperative view showing the aspect of the clitoral region; note the formed wall of the clitoral prepuce. (**d**) (bottom right): Result 2½ months after reconstruction, note the still reddish colored clitoral tip, turning into brownish with time, and the well defined preputial wall

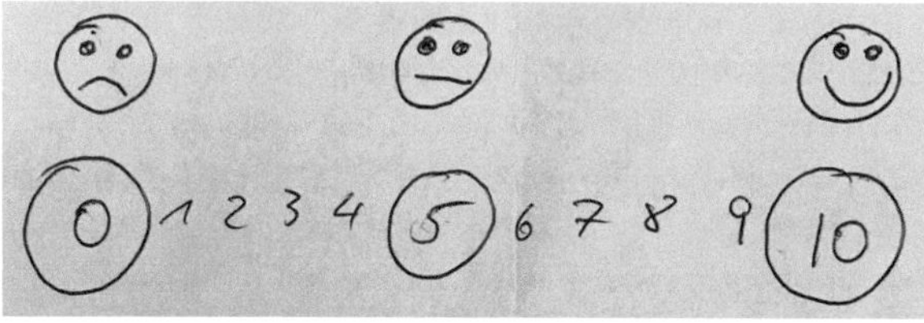

Fig. 3.12 Abstraction scale for clitoral perception (*the very first and original handfree drawing/sketch from the author presented to a patient*). Scale from 0 to 10 as the minimum-maximum value, corresponding to a sad and happy smiley; 5 to declare an average value corresponding to an indifferent smiley

clitoral tip resembling the clitoral glans to cumulate and likewise increase sensory capacity of the clitoral organ. The third is creation of a clitoral prepuce to enhance the form of the anterior vulva and support for mechanic protection of the newly formed clitoral glans.

3.3.2 Vulvar Reconstruction with the Anterior Obturator Artery Perforator Flap (aOAP Flap)

Key attributes for the reconstruction of vulvar units and subunits are symmetry, soft, and pliable tissue showing minor fat, and handling of the vulva as an aesthetic unit. The aOAP flap—acronym for "anterior obturator artery perforator" flap—invented by the author in 2010 [7] and described in the following does unite all these features and some more in order to create an anatomically normal outer female genital following ablative procedures.

3.3.2.1 General Perspective

Vulvar tissue usually shows exceptional flexibility and may therefore lead to the assumption that primary closure even of extended vulvar defects should be sufficient from a practical point of view. However, the conclusion that primary closure of extended vulvar defects is anatomically sufficient does not fit. Primary closure following relevant tissue loss at least leads to tension. Tension leads to deformation, physical discomfort, and functional disorder.

Adequate replacement of the lost tissue instead can support normal anatomy likewise restoring lost tissue properties. A reconstructive approach therefore should be favored compared to primary closure. The result then should be clearly preferable and much more beneficial for the patient. Inadequate tissue transfer instead may frequently lead to other problems such as an excessive vulvar size, unnatural vulvar projection, deformation, and impaired vulvar function.

There are many flaps available for vulvar reconstruction, each showing its own benefits and drawbacks [8–13]. Progress in the knowledge of angiosomes and the design and the composition of flaps leads to an increasing ability to use more ideal tissues tailored to the recipient side and likewise minimize morbidity of the harvest side. Especially pedicled perforator flaps are generally accepted to show favorable results [7, 11, 12]. Perforator flaps evolve as the *gold standard* in reconstructive surgery of diverse regions including the vulva. The aOAP flap is such a pedicled perforator flap [7]. The aOAP flap shows exceptional characteristics for anatomic reconstruction of the vulva, even though the complex anatomy of the vulva will almost always be simplified by reconstructive procedures to a certain extent. Nevertheless, aOAP-flap vulvar reconstruction shows many outstanding benefits. For example, the aOAP flap is located nearby the vulva and thereby optimizes the operative setting; it is of less subcutaneous tissue, it is dissected as a pedicled fasciocutaneous island flap, it is vascularized by a true umbrellalike perforator vessel originating from the obturator artery and vein, harvest side is closed primarily, and the recipient side can be treated as an aesthetic unit. Moreover, closure of the harvest side is done as in medial thigh lifts, resulting in inconspicuous scarring and favorable contour. Additionally, due to the minor subcutaneous tissue found at the genitofemoral sulcus, the aOAP flap is thin and pliable providing a more anatomically normal haptic and contour of the reconstructed vulva. Another major benefit of the aOAP flap is that it provides an adequate mobility for locoregional, tension-free, and tunneled transposition due to mobility of the skeletonized pedicle. Moreover, the flap is moldable due to a direct umbrellalike course of the aOAP perforator vessel to the subdermal plexus allowing for subcutaneous thinning in periphery to the subcutaneous entry of the pedicle. In particular, reconstruction of the region of the vestibule profits from the before-mentioned characteristics provided by an islanded and tunneled aOAP flap. Sensory supply from the obturator nerve usually paralleling the pedicle can be included in the flap and even that from the pudendal nerve when encountered during dissection. The latter leads to a neurovascular tissue transfer optimizing the reconstructive result for the patient.

Unlike both the pudendal thigh flap [14], partly harvested from the same region as the aOAP flap, and the lotus petal flap harvested from the gluteal crease [15, 16], the aOAP flap is not dependent on a lipocutaneous or subcutaneous stalk harboring its blood supply and likewise restricting the capability of flap transposition. Branches of the internal pudendal artery and vein provide blood supply of the pudendal thigh flap and lotus petal flap. The aOAP flap instead obtaining its blood supply by a true perforator originating from the obturator artery and vein can be dissected as an island flap likewise lifting its characteristics out of those of other flaps available for locoregional vulvar reconstruction.

The outer female genital is one of the most sensitive areas of human beings. A substantial decrease in visible and deforming scarring is therefore desirable. Comparing the harvest side of the aOAP flap with other regional pedicled perforator flaps for vulvar reconstruction, there is no other showing similar characteristics for inconspicuous scarring even though also other tunneled options are available [11, 12].

However, as I mentioned beforehand each flap has two sides and the aOAP flap does also. As described beforehand the aOAP flap has many benefits, but on the other hand it is not easy to do. So, it needs time and advanced microsurgical skills to adapt the flap procedure. Regarding dissection, the small caliber of the aOAP pedicle is also a clear drawback and needs experience in perforator dissection. Identification of the small calibered aOAP pedicle on the most proximal surface of the gracilis aponeurosis is initially quite easy to perform, but dissection of the vulnerable pedicle through and beyond the aponeurosis and the underlying muscle is clearly challenging and somewhat time consuming. Nevertheless, it is critical to do that, because the pedicle needs mobility. Loop magnification 4.0× or higher and fine instruments for microsurgical dissection are essential. The deeper the dissection continues a more complex vascular and neural network is encountered. Dissection of the pedicle should be done nearby its origin to gain enough mobility of the flap for tension-free transposition. As a consequence, performing an aOAP flap needs both experience in microsurgical perforator dissection and adequate microsurgical instruments/equipment.

Even though the aOAP flap is not easy to dissect, it is still the thinnest pedicled flap being made available for vulvar reconstruction. Finally, reconstructive potential in detail depends on the individual anatomic conditions found in the remaining vulva. The reconstructive result that can be achieved with aOAP flap is outstanding compared with the reconstructive potentials of other flap techniques described until now.

3.3.2.2 The aOAP Flap Procedure (Video 3.2)

Consider that anatomic reconstruction of the vulva should almost always be symmetric. That means a both-sided vulvar defect is best handled with an also both-sided aOAP-flap design. Even though a one-sided flap crossing the midline at the anterior or posterior commissure might be sufficient in terms of tissue replacement it usually does not fit in terms of anatomy. FGM/C type III patients almost always show both-sided tissue loss requiring symmetric aOAP-flap reconstruction (Fig. 3.13). Other acquired deformities may be unilateral (see Fig. 1.18) or bilateral (Fig. 3.14) in origin as in perineal lacerations following episiotomy, or resection of malignancies and Bartholin's cyst. In such one-sided vulvar defects a one-sided flap design should be mostly adequate, of course.

Before starting the procedure precise evaluation of the vulva is necessary. All absent anatomic details should be defined and conceptually included in the entire reconstructive plan to restore form and function of the vulva.

The patient then is placed in the lithotomy position and marked on the skin according to the regular vascular anatomy, which is of vital importance to the survival of the flap. Localizing the gracilis muscle and the inferior pubic ramus is important for planning of the flap procedure. The anterior obturator artery perforator (aOAP) is classified as constant [7]. The aOAP flap therefore proves its suitability and versatility in the reconstruction of vulvar defects. Emergence of the aOAP vessel close to the inferior pubic ramus usually half way of the transverse diameter of the aponeurosis of the gracilis muscle is localized with an audible Doppler probe and marked on the skin. A crescent-shaped or fusiform skin island is designed slightly decentralized over the detected perforator and its axis parallel to the genitofemoral sulcus on both sides or only the left or the right

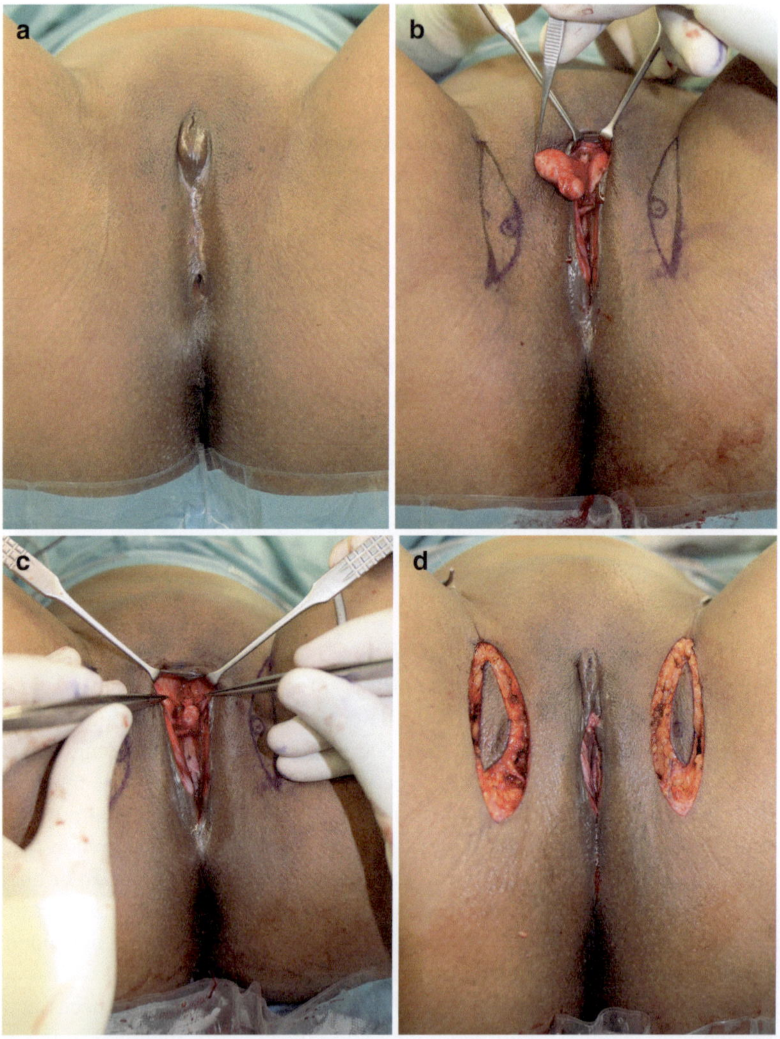

Fig. 3.13 Reconstruction of the vulva in a 25-year-old woman showing a FGM/C type III deformity and a distinct cyst of the clitoral stump. (**a**) (top left) Preoperative view showing the FGM/C type III amputated upper and middle third of the vulva with a subtotal closure of vestibule and absence of the clitoral glans; note the mass in the region of the clitoris representing a cyst of the clitoral stump. (**b**) (top right) Intraoperative view showing dissection of the clitoral bodies including the clitoral cyst following opening of the vestibule and adjusted OD-flap incision; the both-sided aOAP flaps are already marked on the skin for later reconstruction of the vestibule. (**c**) (middle left) Intraoperative view following excision of the clitoral cyst and isolation of the clitoral stump; microsurgical dissection of the clitoral nerves is almost accomplished ready for reconstruction of the clitoral tip with the NMCS procedure. (**d**) (middle right) Intraoperative view after microsurgical reconstruction of the clitoral tip with the NMCS procedure, prepuce reconstruction with an adjusted OD flap, and completed harvest of both-sided aOAP flaps before tunneled transposition of each. (**e**) (bottom left) Intraoperative view at rest after reconstruction has been done. (**f**) (bottom right) Final result showing the aOAP-formed vestibule, the newly formed clitoral tip, the created prepuce, and the vaginal introitus with the region of the hymen

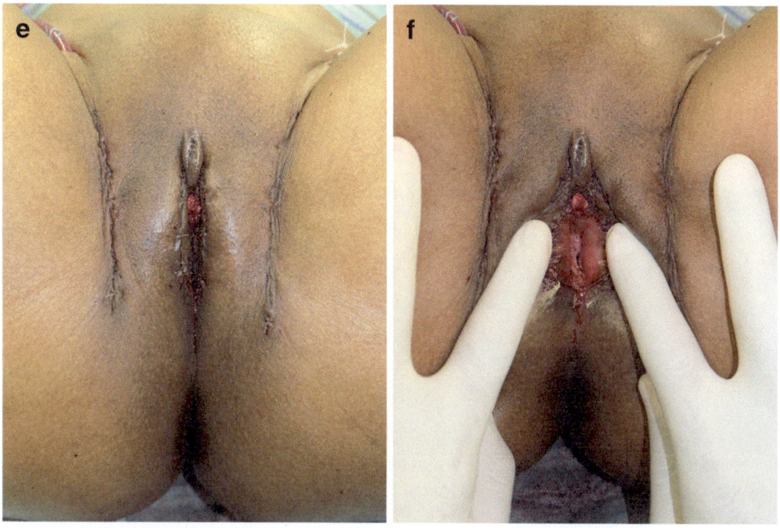

Fig. 3.13 (continued)

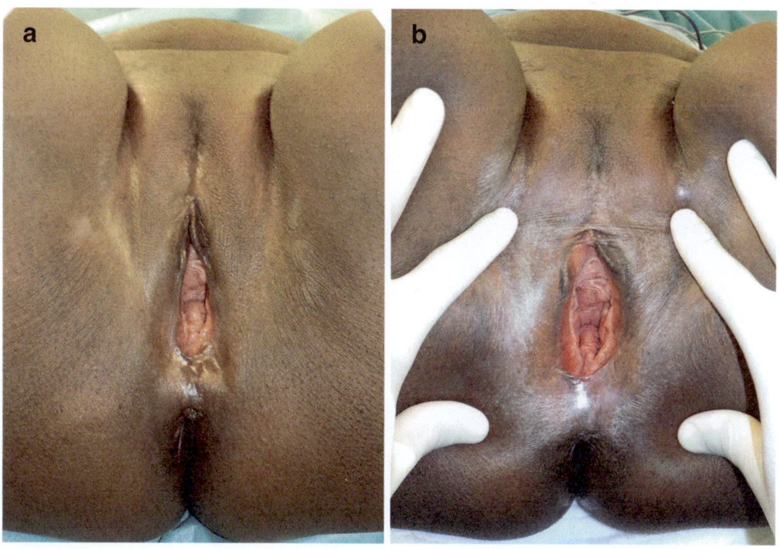

Fig. 3.14 Reconstruction of the vulva in a 35-year-old woman with a both-sided vulvar deformity following perineal rupture during delivery suffering from pain and an open introitus. (**a**) (top left) Preoperative view at rest showing the widened posterior commissure and the perineal scar accentuated to the right. (**b**) (top right) Preoperative view showing the complex perineal scar extending toward the posterior vaginal wall. (**c**) (middle left) Intraoperative view following excision of the scar, harvest, and transposition of the aOAP flaps prior to wound closure. (**d**) (middle right) Intraoperative view at rest after inset of the aOAP flaps interlocking at the posterior commissure; note the normalized and stable posterior commissure. (**e**) (bottom left) Intraoperative view after reconstruction showing the vestibule and the vaginal introitus; note the retracted scar of the posterior vaginal introitus. (**f**) (bottom right) Final result in the upright position; note the normal silhouette of the vulva and the genitofemoral sulcus

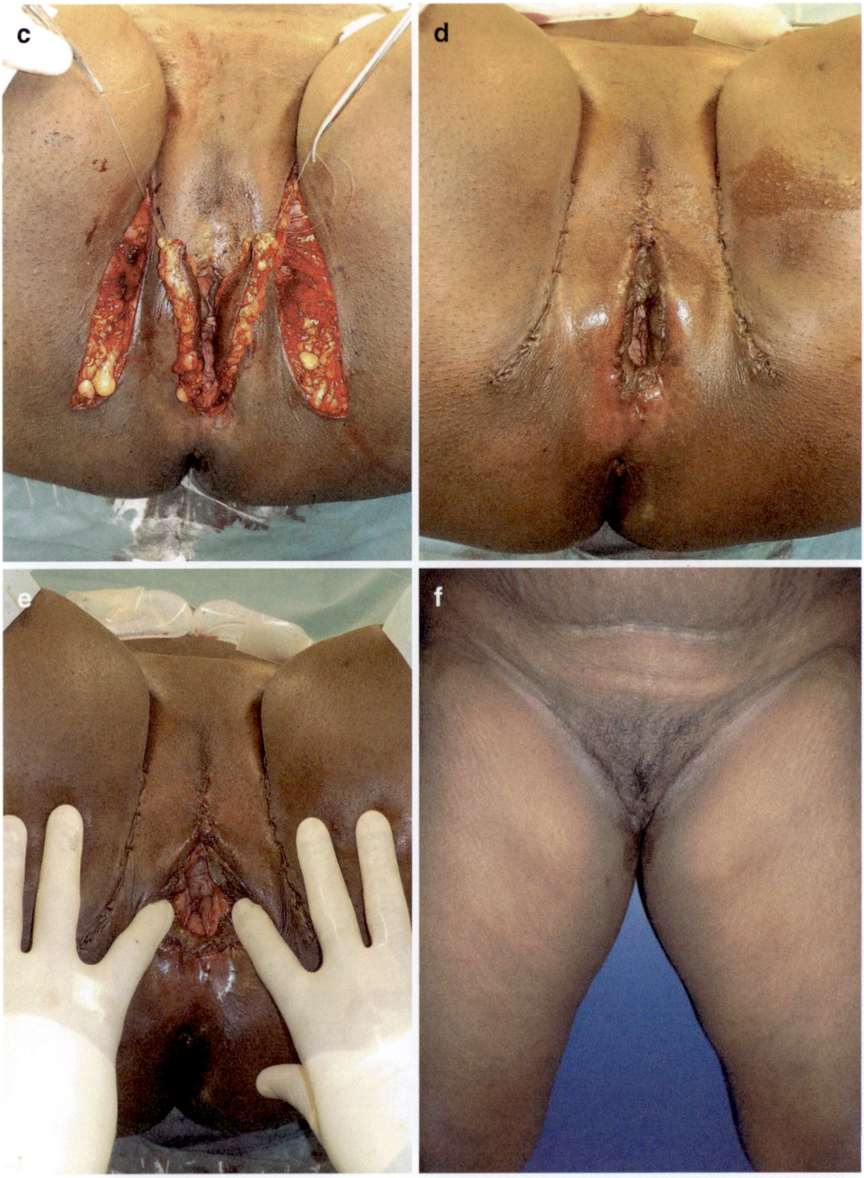

Fig. 3.14 (continued)

side depending on the reconstructive needs. Despite the axis, symmetry of the flap can be adjusted according to both size and shape of the vulvar defect. As shown later de-epithelializing and/or splitting of the aOAP flap is also possible to adapt to the reconstructive needs. Bilaterally designed aOAP flaps prepared to coalesce sagittally encircling the vaginal introitus are usually planned to address bilateral vulvar defects.

Due to the angiosome of the aOAP vessel [7], the size of the flap can be set up to 7 [cm] in width and 15 [cm] in length from the anterior border of the M. adductor longus muscle to the posterior border of the adductor magnus muscle. Incision starts at the anterior-most part of the flap localized on the level of the M. adductor longus and continues all the way down and through the fascia lata. Consolidation of the fascia with the skin by using a fascio-dermal single-knot stitch with a 5.0 absorbable or nonabsorbable monofilament suture eases dissection and secures the skin from being sheared off while dissection. This suture can also be used to support the flap while dissecting. Elevation of the flap proceeds subfascially from anterolateral to posteromedial extending to the anterior border of the aponeurosis of the gracilis muscle. Attention must now be paid to carefully identify the aOAP pedicle on surface or at the posterior border of the aponeurosis of the gracilis muscle situated close to the inferior pubic ramus.

In case of a musculocutaneous [7] course of the aOAP pedicle the aponeurosis and gracilis muscle are split according to fiber direction to allow for both primary visualization of the pedicle and secondary sliding of the pedicle during transposition of the aOAP flap. Dissection of the pedicle is continued, usually down to the anterior branch of the obturator artery, to obtain a maximum of mobility for subsequent tension-free transposition of the flap.

In case of a septocutaneous [7] course of the aOAP pedicle the aponeurosis of the gracilis muscle is divided over a short distance perpendicular to fiber direction to allow for both primary visualization and dissection of the pedicle and secondary shifting of the pedicle during transposition of the aOAP flap.

It is important to be aware that dissection of the small calibered pedicle is difficult. The deeper the dissection progresses a more complex vascular and neural network is encountered. Therefore, the vascular network is susceptible to damage resulting from dissection. Ramifications of the muscle must be clipped and cut through carefully to free the pedicle.

When the pedicle is adequately visualized, incision of the entire skin island can then be completed to finally raise the flap. The posterior border of the flap is determined by the region of the adductor magnus muscle that is posterior to the pedicle. Posterior to the pedicle dissection plane changes from deep to superficial. Attention to this transition zone is important to exclude the fatty tissue bulk in the region of the gluteo-femoral crease, which continues with the genitofemoral sulcus. The deep fascia or fascia lata and the superficial fascia or Colles' fascia anatomically reflect this zone of transition. The investing fascia of the major labias also mirroring the Colles' fascia determines the medial border of the flap.

In case of extensive vulvoperineal defects, the dimension of the flap can be escalated per side to 7 cm in width and 15 cm in length. The larger the skin island, the more it may profit from an additional vein. However, the main pedicle is the most important one and is therefore objectified preoperatively by a Doppler probe and marked on the skin. An additional vein might be detected intraoperatively. If such a superficial vein is encountered at the medial border of the flap it might be included to support vasculature. It is important, however, that an additional vein does not tend to block mobility of the pedicle or the entire flap, respectively.

When the aOAP flap is stalked solely on its mobilized pedicle, freed of any subcutaneous attachments, it is ready for transposition. Tunnels are then made for subcutaneous transposition connecting the harvest side with the recipient side. For this purpose subcutaneous dissection starts at the vestibular border on the side of the defect all the way to the harvest side. Meticulous hemostasis must be done to rule out later tunnel hematoma potentially comprising the pedicle while putting vasculature of the aOAP flap into danger. Diameter of the tunnels should be generously made to guaranty for unimpaired passing of the flap and compression-free positioning of the pedicle.

After passing the aOAP flaps tension free through the tunnels right into the defect of the recipient site, the donor site is closed multilayered in terms of a medial thigh lift. Before wound closure soft silicon drains, like Jackson-Pratt Drains, are inserted at the harvest sites. Then the genitofemoral sulcus is recreated by tacking the edge of the fascia lata both sides down to the inferior pubic ramus. For this maneuver I prefer using nonabsorbable braided 0.0 sutures to guaranty for prolonged tensile strength. Due to the fact that the course of the pedicle is nearby the inferior ramus of the pubic bone, tacking of the fascia lata must be performed with great attention to avoid any mechanical impairment of the pedicle. However, all patients felt some inconvenience postoperatively in the region of the inferior pubic ramus resulting from periosteal pexy of the fascia lata. These complaints completely resolve within 3 months postoperatively whereas the recreated contour of the sulcus genitofemoralis persists while equally improving self-image of the patients. Reliable pexy of the fascia lata, therefore, is of utmost importance to complete the aOAP procedure.

Wound closure then is continued three-layered with resorbable monofilament suture material including the Colles' fascia, the subcutaneous layer, and the intracutaneous layer. Suturing should be performed watertight intended to reduce the risk of both maceration and bacterial invasions.

A urinary catheter is placed and usually removed within 3–5 days postoperatively, until full mobilization has been achieved. Sterile dressing is done with antibacterial ointment on the suture line and estrogen ointment within the vaginal introitus.

The patient is confined to bed postoperatively for 48 h with the thighs comfortably abducted on pillows in an effort to avoid tension and/or pressure on the pedicle, the genitofemoral suture line, or the vestibule. Failure of the suture line will most likely lead to an impaired result. The patient is encouraged to keep that position while bedding until sufficient healing and reduced swelling occur—usually within 5–8 days. On day 3 after surgery, however, the patient is mobilized out of bed and the urinary catheter is removed rapidly.

Vaginal discharge must be addressed by daily wound dressings and if necessary by application of antimicrobial suppositories.

In certain cases, usually others than FGM/C involving the perineum, a protective anus praeter might be beneficial to prevent adverse effects of defecation. Generally, adequate preoperative laxatives and postoperative diets for 3–5 days are sufficient in avoiding wound irritations resulting from excretions. Adequate wound healing following vulvoperineal reconstruction largely depends on evading postoperative maceration and/or infection of the suture line causing wound dehiscence, tissue loss, and increased scarring.

3.3.2.3 Advanced Vulvar Reconstruction with the aOAP Flap: The Split-aOAP Flap Technique

In selected cases with eligible tissue conditions the aOAP flap can technically be pushed further always staying on the cutting edge of vulvar reconstruction. Due to the vascular anatomy of the aOAP flap it is capable to be split transdermally, so its skin island can be more tailored to the tissue needs of the vulvar vestibule. Local tissue of the vestibule like the roots of the minor labias or minor labias that have been recreated from local tissue remnants can be used and included within the flap design for more sophisticated anatomic creations. It is possible thereby to create minor labias partially or completely combined with the reconstruction of the vestibule. Meticulous microsurgical preparation with magnifying loupes is crucial. However, immediate (Fig. 3.15) and long-term (Fig. 3.16) results are excellent.

Planning of the procedure must be done properly followed by precise dissection of the split aOAP flaps (Fig. 3.17). Incisions through the cutis and the dermal layer should be made while tightening of the skin (Fig. 3.17d). Once reaching the subdermal plexus, further loosening of the skin islands is performed in a blunt spreading manner keeping vessel arcades intact while weakening connective tissue septa and bands. After aOAP-flap splitting is completed, the skin paralleling the introitus is prepared to resemble minor labias. When I do reconstruction of the minor labias with tissue of the midline I usually create a both-sided anteriorly based flap of the skin and scar flanking the introitus (Fig. 3.17d). These skin areas arise following median opening of the introitus in FGM/C type III patients (see Fig. 3.15b). After lifting the minor labia flaps up they are fixed with subcutaneous single-knot sutures to form a vertical brick. They are mostly posteriorly detached from the underground so they can be integrated in the split aOAP flaps later. Region of detachment, however, depends on the intended flap planning. It is essential then that the minor labia flap is positioned in between the angled legs of the aOAP flap. So the aOAP flap can recreate the introitus on both sides of the vestibulum.

In my opinion the described split-aOAP flap technique offers perfect results but is clearly more challenging to dissect as the standard aOAP flap and therefore harder to perform. A certain level of experience with the flap is required to handle dissection. You should be aware that vasculature is the limiting factor and it must be

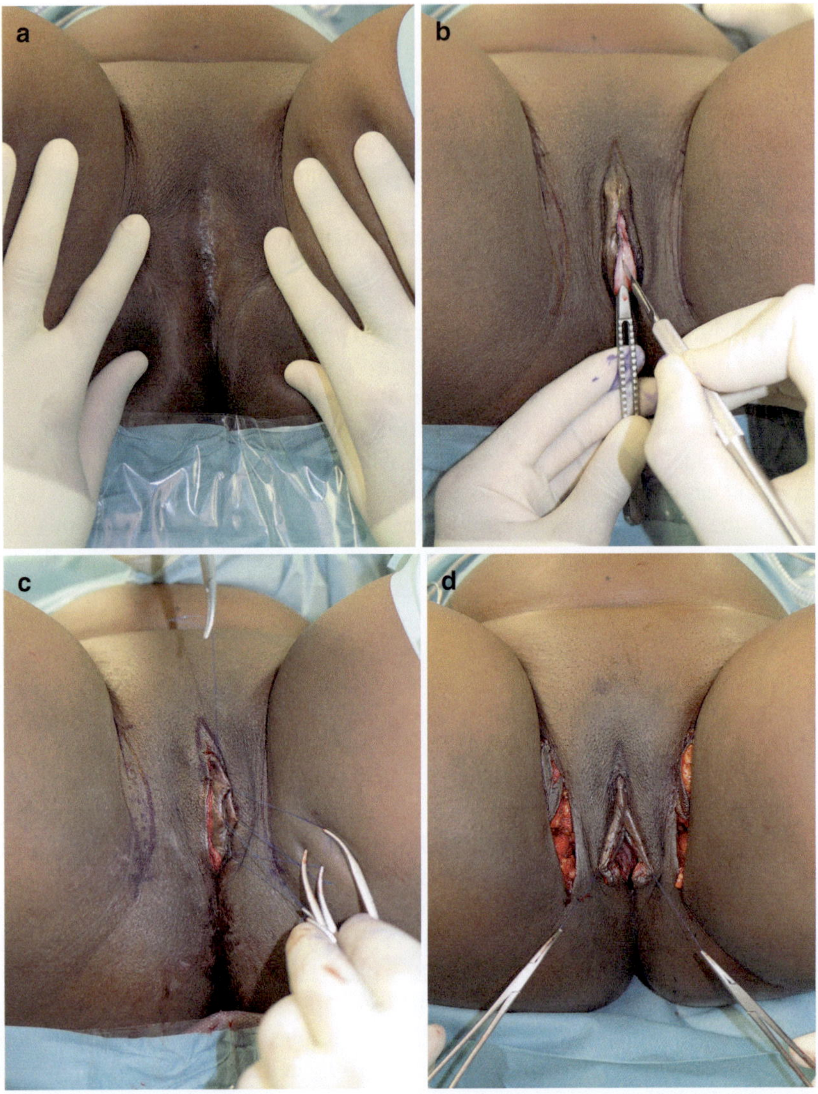

Fig. 3.15 Reconstruction of the vulva in a 26-year-old woman showing a FGM/C type III deformity with adjustable tissue in the region of the midline. (**a**) (top left) Preoperative view of the infibulated outer genital showing subtotal closure of the vestibule. (**b**) (top right) Intraoperative view showing the opening of the vestibule; the anterior border of the vestibule must be determined beforehand; I prefer a clear cut with a knife performed on smooth and plane instrument to protect the vestibular skin and the urethral orifice; infiltration of a local anesthetic with adrenalin eases the procedure. (**c**) (middle left) Intraoperative view showing the molded minor labias out off the vestibular skin. (**d**) (middle right) Intraoperative view after completing harvest of the aOAP flaps tailored to integrate the preformed minor labias. (**e**) (bottom left) Intraoperative view at rest after reconstruction has been completed; note the natural aspect of the vulva. (**f**) (bottom right) Intraoperative view under slight tension given to the major labias opening the vestibule; note the skin of the aOAP flaps flanking the created minor labias at both the inner and the outer parts

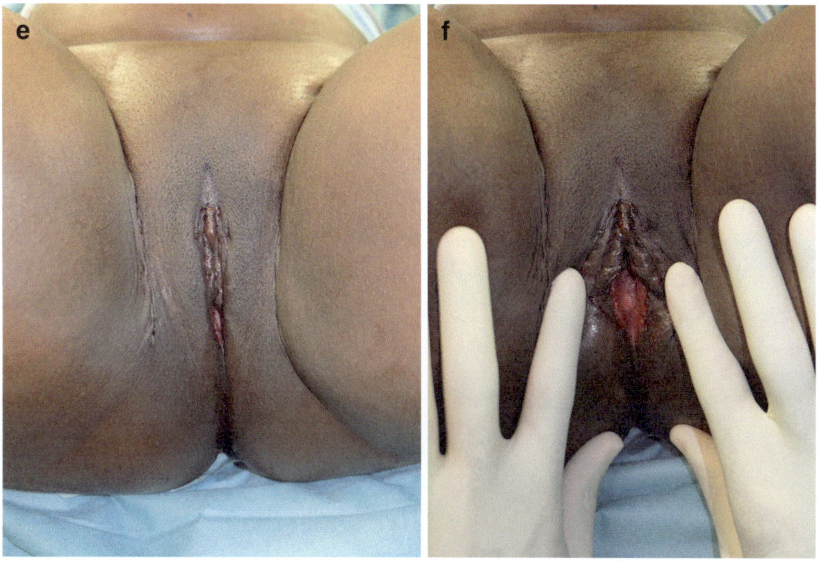

Fig. 3.15 (continued)

preserved. If there is any doubt to guaranty for blood supply, for example due to a particularly small caliber of the aOAP pedicle, you should stay on the safe side and get a reasonable result rather than a highly sophisticated one.

3.3.2.4 Full Vulvar Reconstruction After Vulvectomy (Video 3.3)

Primarily addressing all anatomic details following vulvectomy is a major challenge due to heterogeneity of the vulvar tissue and the homogeneity of the transplanted tissue. However, it is important to create an anatomical result and the aOAP flap offers the best conditions from the viewpoint of reconstruction (Fig. 3.18). Surgically curing lichen sclerosus et atrophicus on an advanced stage of the disease exemplarily leaves an extremely complex defect comprising the prepuce, sometimes skin of the clitoral tip, roots of minor labias and minor labias itself, the reflecting fold of the minor and major labias, the major labias, and last but not least skin of the inner vestibule located in between the clitoral tip and the orifice of the urethra as well as the skin in between the hymen and the posterior commissure (Fig. 3.18c). The aOAP flaps then need to be arranged by suturing that way that they do reflect a three-dimensional anatomic reconstruction rather than a two-dimensional defect closure. That is in the end the difficulty of reconstruction (Fig. 3.18e, f).

3.3.2.5 Reconstruction in FGM Type IV

FGM type IV is very heterogeneous in detail and therefore often provides with unexpected findings and conditions such as tear down of the anterior labial roots in an attempt to forcibly discipline women. Reconstructive needs may range from simple to complex but do usually exclude larger tissue transfers.

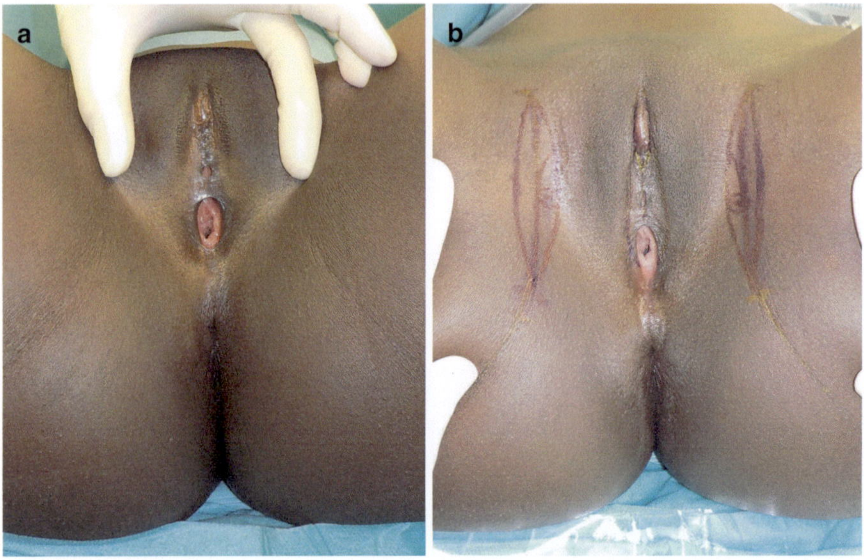

Fig. 3.16 Reconstruction of the vulva in a 20-year-old woman showing a FGM/C type III deformity with adjustable tissue in the region of the midline. (**a**) (rooftop left) Preoperative view at rest showing absence of the clitoral tip, prepuce, minor labias, und subtotal closure of the vestibule. (**b**) (rooftop right) Preoperative view under slight tension of the genitofemoral skin; note the markings of the leaf-shaped aOAP flaps; the anterior medial parts will be removed later while the remaining flap is split transdermally into halves to fit in with the later vestibular arrangement. (**c**) (top left) Intraoperative view after opening of the vestibule and microsurgical preparation of the clitoral stump on the level of the deep clitoral bodies; the clitoral nerves are already dissected ready for the neurotization of the clitoral stump (NMCS procedure). (**d**) (top right) Intraoperative view showing procedure of molding of the inner vestibular unit resembling the region of the minor labias. (**e**) (middle left) Intraoperative view after completion of forming of the inner vestibule and dissection of the aOAP flaps; note that the upper medial part of the right aOAP flap was already removed prior to the splitting procedure as it will be done on the left side; note the fine tip of the clitoris within the anterior vestibule immediately positioned under the newly formed prepuce. (**f**) (middle right) Intraoperative view after completion of reconstruction; note the relaxed aspect of both the vestibule and the vaginal introitus; the newly formed clitoral tip has to be positioned low within the anterior vestibule due to the amputation level located at the first third of the clitoral bodies. (**g**) (bottom left) Postoperative view at rest 1 year after reconstruction; note the normal aspect of the outer vulva and inconspicuous scars of both the vulva and the harvest side. (**h**) (bottom right) Final result 1 year after reconstruction with slight tension given to the genitofemoral skin; note the normalized anatomic details of the inner vestibule; the clitoral tip is re-epithelialized. (**i**) (basement left) Final result 1 year postoperatively in the upright position; note the overall natural characteristic of the vulvar silhouette

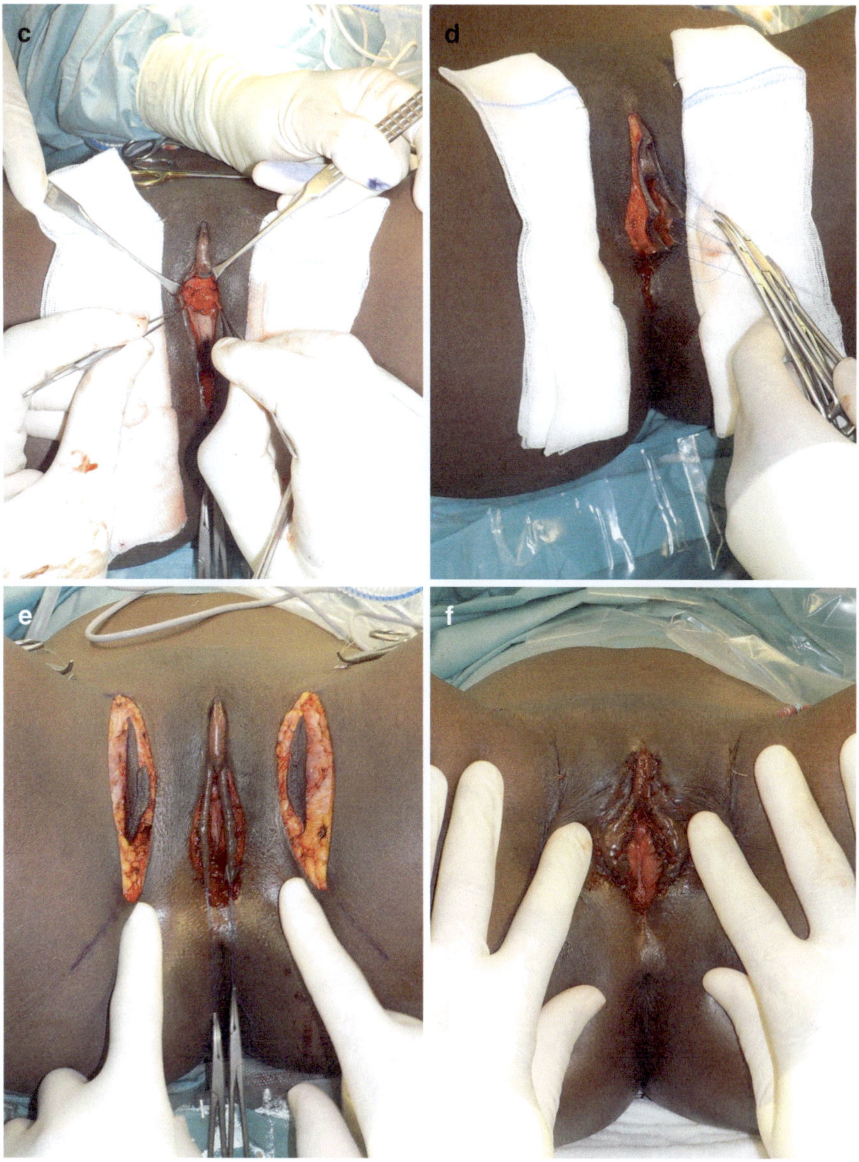

Fig. 3.16 (continued)

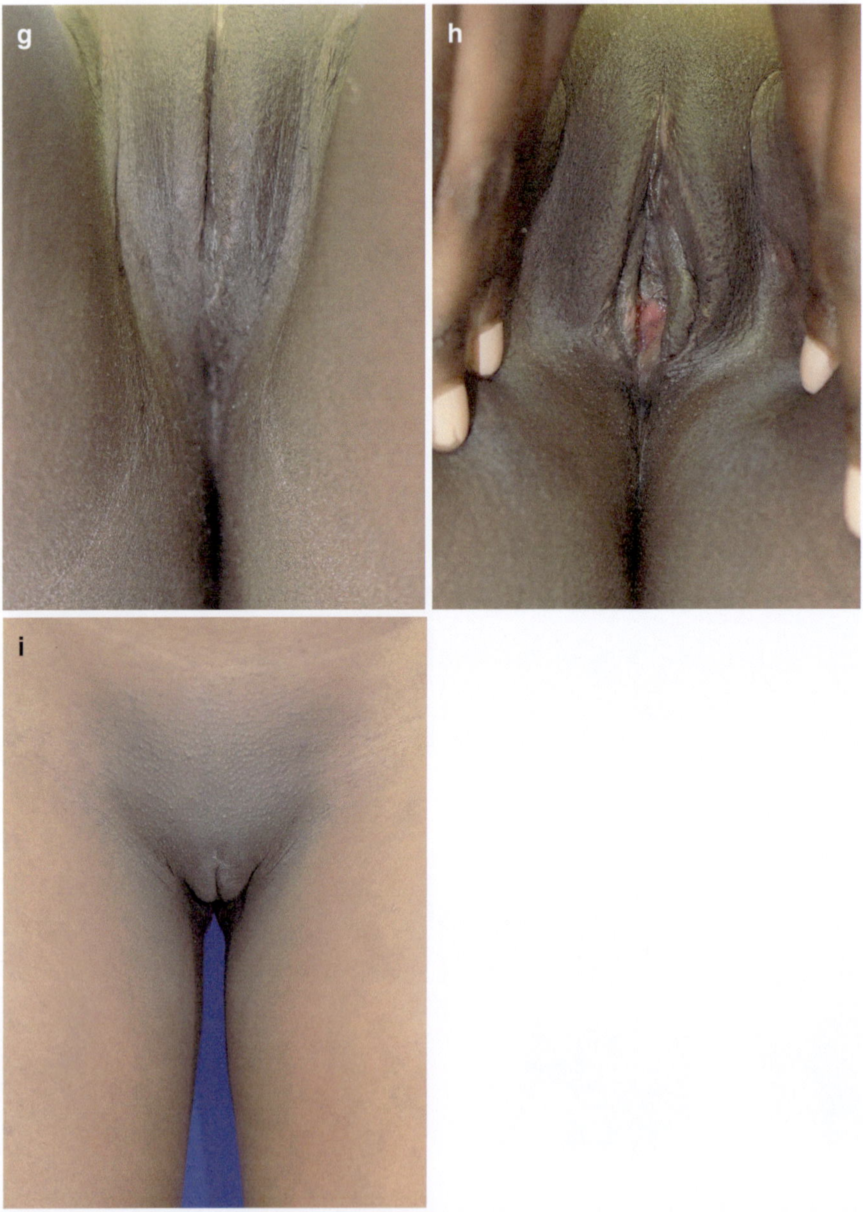

Fig. 3.16 (continued)

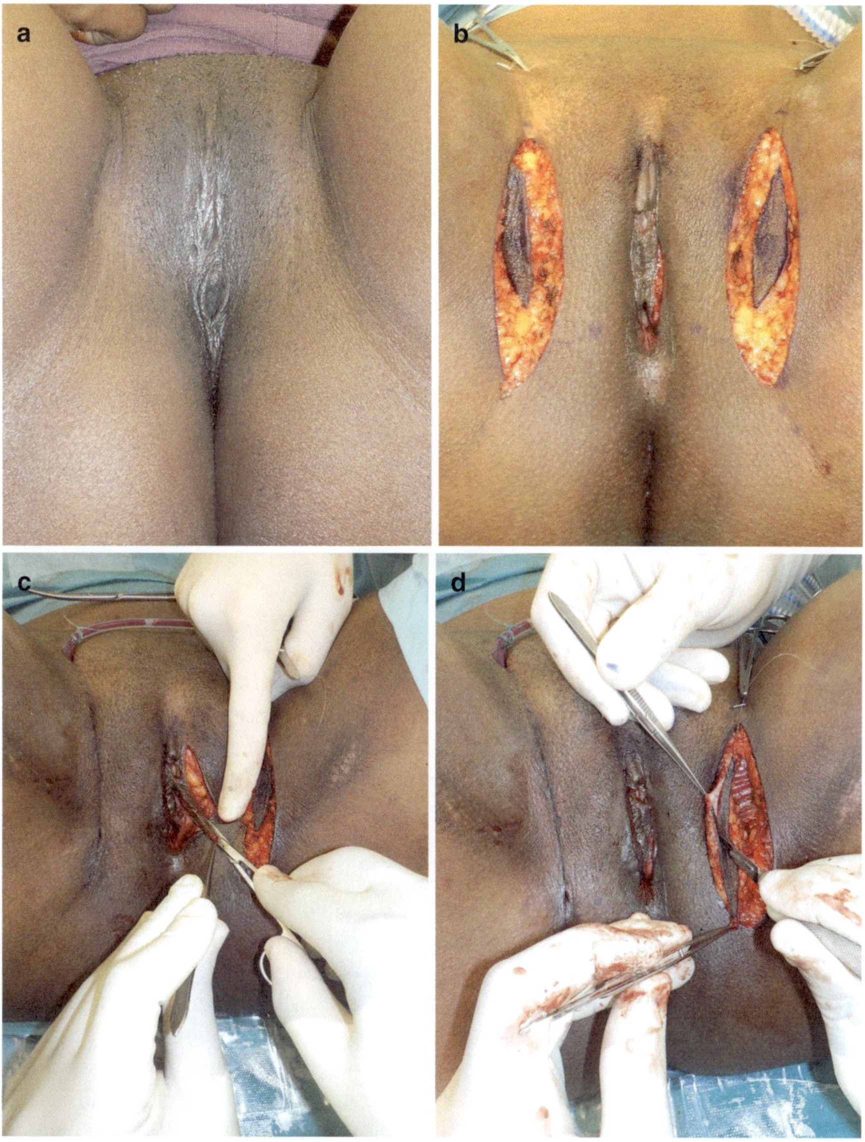

Fig. 3.17 Reconstruction of the vulva in a 19-year-old woman presenting with a FGM/C type III deformity and adjustable tissue in the region of the midline. (**a**) (top left) Preoperative view at rest showing the infibulated outer genital with subtotal closure of the vestibule. (**b**) (top right) Intraoperative view showing harvest of the aOAP flaps prior to the splitting maneuver; the vestibule was already opened. (**c**) (middle left) Intraoperative view showing the splitting maneuver of the left aOAP flap; incision is made while tightening of the flap. (**d**) (middle right) Intraoperative view demonstrating posterior detachment of the anteriorly stalked minor labia flap of the left-sided vestibule. (**e**) (bottom left) Intraoperative view after reconstruction has been completed showing the vestibule and the vaginal introitus. (**f**) (bottom right) Final result 1 year after surgery; in the upright position; note the anatomical normal silhouette of the vulva and the genitofemoral sulcus

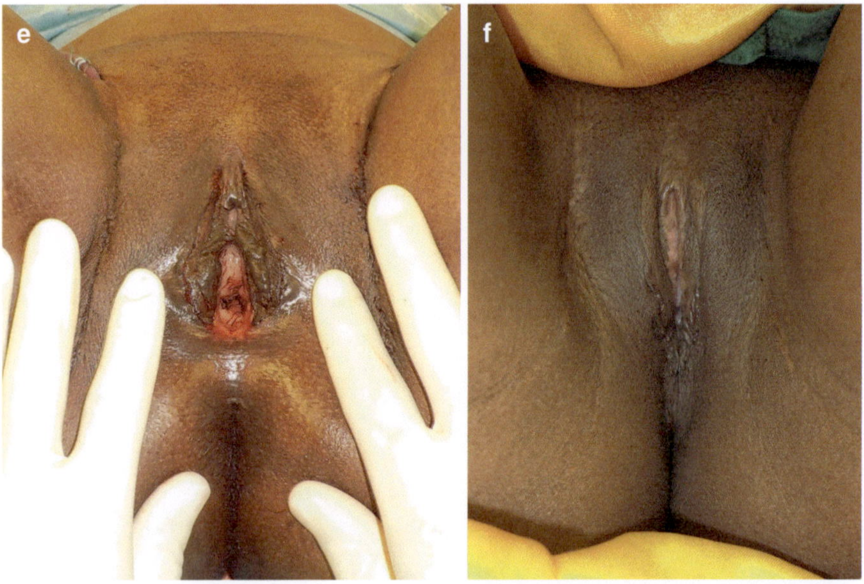

Fig. 3.17 (continued)

3.3.2.6 Algorithm for Complex Vulvar Reconstruction

Initial evaluation of the underlying tissue defects is necessary to bring out all anatomic problems. The sum of deficits lastly assigns the needs for reconstruction. Evaluation is started in the region of the prepuce, followed by deep palpation of the clitoral organ remained, assessment of the lost tissue of the minor and major labias, followed by general exploration of the vulvar vestibule. Furthermore assessment of scars, clitoral cysts, asymmetries, tissue conditions, hair distribution, skin quality, and overall anatomic impression are identified. While working on these details the surgeon is able to form a visual reconstructive composition in his/her mind.

Based on the described techniques in this book, a three-staged algorithm can be used to stepwise implement the reconstructive needs. In the different degrees of FGM/C patients there are generally three key problems regarding tissue loss. The first is loss of the clitoral prepuce found in FGM/C type I, II, and III. The second is partial loss of the clitoral organ potentially found in FGM/C type I and usually faced in FGM/C type II, and III. The third is varying loss of the vulvar vestibule including minor and major labias met in FGM/C type II, and especially type III.

The anterior region of the vulva is best addressed with the OD flap offering a generous surgical approach to the clitoral organ while providing a fine flap concept to recreate the prepuce (see Sect. 3.2.2). The NMCS procedure then offers optimized conditions enabling for reinnervation of the newly formed clitoral tip (see Sect. 3.2.3). Finally the aOAP flap then provides an advanced technical capability for symmetrical recreation of the lost tissue of the vulva including the vestibule (see Sect. 3.3). These three techniques lastly form the three-staged algorithm mentioned above and listed in Table 3.1.

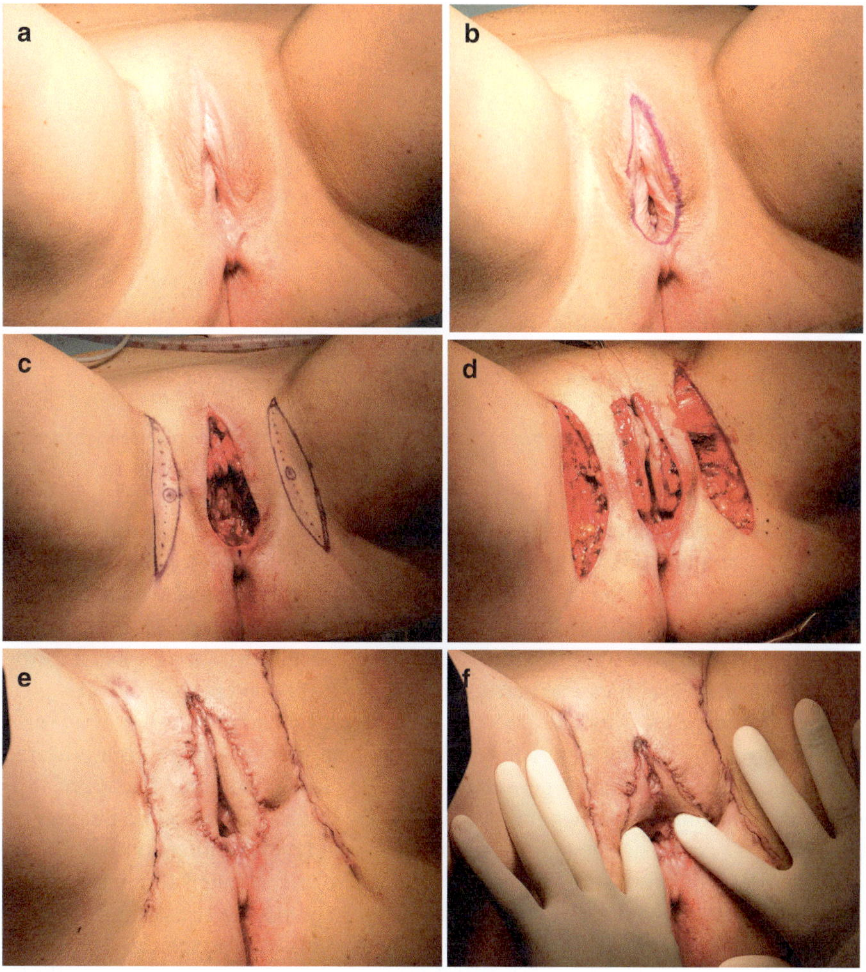

Fig. 3.18 Full vulvar reconstruction in a 40-year-old woman following excision of lichen sclerosus et atrophicus. (**a**) (top left) Preoperative view showing the atrophic and coalesced vulvar vestibule. (**b**) (top right) Preoperative view after marking of the incision line; note that skin of the outer and inner vulvar will extensively be removed. (**c**) (middle left) Intraoperative view demonstrating the extended vulvar defect and markings of the both-sided aOAP-flap incision line; note the exocentric position of the perforator entering the subcutis of the flaps. (**d**) (middle right) Intraoperative view after tunneled transposition of the both-sided aOAP flap into the vestibule. (**e**) (bottom left) Intraoperative view at rest after finishing the reconstructive procedure; note that the anterior-most part of the aOAP flap was tailored by using a both-sided OD flap technique to form a prepuce; even though the minor labias are lacking, the result conveys normality. (**f**) (bottom right) Intraoperative view of the reconstructed vulva while spreading the vestibule; note that both aOAP flaps encircle the centrally located clitoral tip while filling in the tissue defect in between the outer orifice of the urethra and the lower border of the clitoral tip

Table 3.1 Algorithm for vulvar reconstruction in FGM patients

	Degree of tissue loss				
	FGM I		FGM II	FGM III	FGM IV
Reconstructive procedure	Prepuce	Prepuce and clitoral glans/ corpora	Prepuce and clitoral glans/ corpora and minor labias	Prepuce and clitoral glans/ corpora and minor labias and major labias	Prepuce and clitoral glans/ corpora and minor labias and major labias
OD flap	x	x	x	x	(x)
NMCS		x	x	x	(x)
aOAP flap			(x)	x	(x)

OD flap Omega-Domed flap, *NMCS* Neurotizing and molding of the clitoral stump, *aOAP flap* anterior Obturator artery perforator flap, *FGM* Female genital mutilation, () optionally

3.4 Adjunctives

As with other procedures supplementary measures sometimes effectively support the primary result. Due to the given anatomy hair growth within the vestibule or the vaginal introitus following aOAP-flap vulvar reconstruction may lead to discomfort, dyspareunia, and an allover irritating aspect. Epilation, therefore, is an important and supplementary procedure in case of inevitable transposition of a hair-bearing genitofemoral sulcus. It can be performed preoperatively and postoperatively.

There are different ways for permanent hair removal and a wide variety of technologies available. In my experience permanent hair removal using a high-powered diode laser with a wavelength between 800 and 950 nm, a maximum fluence of 44 J/cm^2, and a maximum wavelength of 12 Hz is one of the most effective treatments. Such systems can easily be tailored to different skin types. Application is comfortable especially by precooling of the treated area with an integrated aluminum probe. When correctly applied side effects are low and may include tweaking sensations during the treatment or short-time erythema afterwards. It is conceivable that thermally induced micro-thrombosis of subdermal capillaries and tissue loss might be an issue, but I never observed such side effects.

Due to different hair growth phases repeated treatments are usually necessary and can be performed in between 6- and 12-week intervals. It might be beneficial, however, to vary the intervals just to address the changing hair cycles.

3.5 Postoperative Care

Concerning my experience patients scheduled for complex vulvar reconstructions are best monitored and supported on an inpatient basis. Immediate postoperative feedback and advice by the surgeon are critical and important for the patient as it provides stability and trust in the gained vulvar capacity. Especially FGM patients frequently show a certain culturally related restraint in handling their outer genital as the integral part of their femininity.

3.5.1 Clitoral and Prepuce Reconstruction

Patients are usually admitted for overnight observation and seen for first follow-up at postoperative day 1. Any problems with hematoma should be obvious by this time. The patient is again informed concerning the operative course and instructed in wound care and general behavior for the next days. The urinary catheter is removed after general instructions have been completed on day 1. Daily cleansing with an appropriate antiseptic agent, application of antibacterial ointment, estrogen crème, and mechanical relief is recommended. Menses are clinically not interfering. After discharge at postoperative day 2 or 3 the next follow-up is *n* days 7–9. Follow-up visits then are typically at 3 weeks, 3 months, 6 months, and 12 months postoperatively. Patients may be released to full activity at 3 weeks and may in selected cases also attempt intercourse then as tolerated. Sexual intercourse, however, is generally not recommended until week 6 postoperatively has been completed. Smoking, of course, should generally be avoided until healing occurs.

3.5.2 Complex Vulvar Reconstruction

Concerning vulvar reconstruction, daily follow-ups from postoperative day 1 to discharge—usually on days 8–10—are performed. Any problems resulting from hematoma, impaired skin/flap viability, or wound infection should have been objectified by this time and likewise effectively handled.

Bed rest in the supine position with the legs slightly spread and padded on pillows is confined for 2 days postoperatively. On day 3, ambulation is permitted. Prolonged compression of the outer genital region by prolonged closing of the legs should be strictly avoided for a minimum of 5 days. In addition, a 10-day supply of decongestant medications is recommended. Local application of moisturized compresses using sodium chloride can ease postoperative swelling. Nevertheless, local application of ice is strictly forbidden as it can bring flap viability into danger. Antibiotics, analgesics, and a stool softener are applied for 8–10 days. Urethral catheter should be left in place until full mobilization has been accomplished, usually on days 3–5. After discharge follow-up visits are typically at 3 weeks, 6 weeks, 6 months, and 12 months postoperatively. Patients may be released to full activity at 6 weeks and may also attempt intercourse then as tolerated. However, extreme load on the outer genital induced by cycling for example might not be tolerated until 3 months postoperatively. Smoking, again, should generally be avoided until healing occurs.

3.6 Management of Complications

Due to several perioperative and postoperative protocols mentioned below complications are rare following vulvar reconstructions. I usually don't see for example infections, hematomas, or even flap necrosis in my patients. However, complications might be generally associated with operative procedures and should therefore be discussed.

3.6.1 General Perspective

As with other surgical interventions, general complications in vulvar reconstruction consist of bleeding, hematoma, swelling, pain, impaired vasculature, or scarring. Special complications consist of the stenosis of the vaginal introitus, or consecutive hair growth on the flaps positioned within the vestibule.

First of all, accurate and less traumatizing surgical techniques are critical and likewise the first step in avoiding perioperative and postoperative complications. In addition, antibiotic prophylaxis and meticulous wound/skin care are recommended to prevent wound infections, maceration, and prolonged wound healing. Due to the close proximity of both vulva and anus antibiotics should be administered that are active against both Gram-positive and Gram-negative anaerobic bacteria commonly found in the vagina and the gut. To cover all these bacteria cephalosporin of fourth generation and metronidazole can be used simultaneously for example.

3.6.2 Primary Complication

3.6.2.1 Pain

In the surgical care pain management is a daily issue. However, physiologically reducing inflammation is the key for pain reduction. Besides systemic pharmacologic treatment and application of local anesthetics in the field of surgery, fine handling of the tissues including microsurgical and layer-specific dissection/closure techniques, fine instruments, meticulous hemostasis, and nontraumatic suture materials can reduce inflammation to a minimum, and likewise effectively support pain relief.

Emotional factors require further consideration. To this concern patient education and information are critical for pain management. Questions like “What do I expect after the operation” shall be clarified in detail beforehand.

Apart from non-pharmacologic pain management, there are multiple options available for pharmacological pain management, of course. Besides direct painkillers, systemic antihistamine and cortisone medications do also contribute to pain relief. If more consistent pain relief is needed, oral morphine is an effective instrument. Detailed information about the location and quality of pain is important to adapt pain control to its needs. Muscular pain from the donor site in the region of the aponeurosis of the gracilis muscle, neuropathic pain in the region of the clitoris, or periosteal pain in the region of the inferior ramus of the pubic bone should be differentiated and explained to the patient.

Nevertheless, concerning the underlying reconstructive procedures, severe postoperative pain is usually not an issue. Medications with nonsteroidal anti-inflammatory drugs (NSAIDs) or paracetamol are mostly sufficient to cover usual minor pain. Additional short-time application of cortisone is often beneficial to support pain management and to further reduce swelling and inflammation.

3.6.2.2 Swelling

To a certain extent swelling almost always occurs following vulva or clitoral reconstruction. Tissue swelling usually fades in between 3 and 5 days postoperatively supported by local and/or systemic decongestant medications. I frequently use an additional cortisone medication in decreasing doses for 3 days postoperatively.

3.6.2.3 Hematoma

In my series up till now hematoma following vulvar reconstruction occurred in less than 1% of patients. The subcutaneous tunnel in the region of the major labias, however, should be generally at risk for bleeding and postoperative hematoma due to lacerations of the venous plexus. The main risks are acute physical compression of the pedicle, and secondary induration of the tissue resulting from resorption. Hematoma may also impair flap viability, and provide discomfort for several days. Significant postoperative hematomas, therefore, should be drained immediately and, if necessary, cleared operatively.

3.6.2.4 Infection

Postoperatively the skin of the vulva is susceptible to infections due to both the wound and the impairment of the protecting environment usually prohibiting colonization with pathogenic bacteria. However, I usually do not see wound infections after clitoral or vulvar reconstruction. Infections are best avoided by a meticulous pre- and postoperative care protocol including single dose of a laxative the day before surgery, antibiotic prophylaxis peri- and postoperatively, local antiseptic agents, and sufficient genital hygiene postoperatively.

There are many bacteria forming the endogenous vulvovaginal microflora, which consists of many different Gram-positive and Gram-negative facultative and obligated anaerobic bacteria. When the vulvovaginal environment is in balance, Lactobacillus species should be the main bacterium. It is wellknown, that bacteria, such as Streptococcus species, *Enterococcus faecalis*, Enterobacter species, *Escherichia coli*, or even Pseudomonas species, are also part of the vulvovaginal microflora in healthy asymptomatic women. Local overload of pathogenic bacteria especially due to contamination by uncontrolled defecation usually causes simple wound maceration and likewise prolonged wound healing. In the rare case that pathogenic bacteria dominate the endogenous microflora while impairing tissues' integrity in the operative field, operative revision is indicated. Labial abscesses can generally occur after any surgical intervention. To rule out the development of serious phlegmonous infections, treatment should include broad-spectrum antibiotics and immediate finding-based surgical interventions. Wound secretion, of course, should be taken for microbiologic examination.

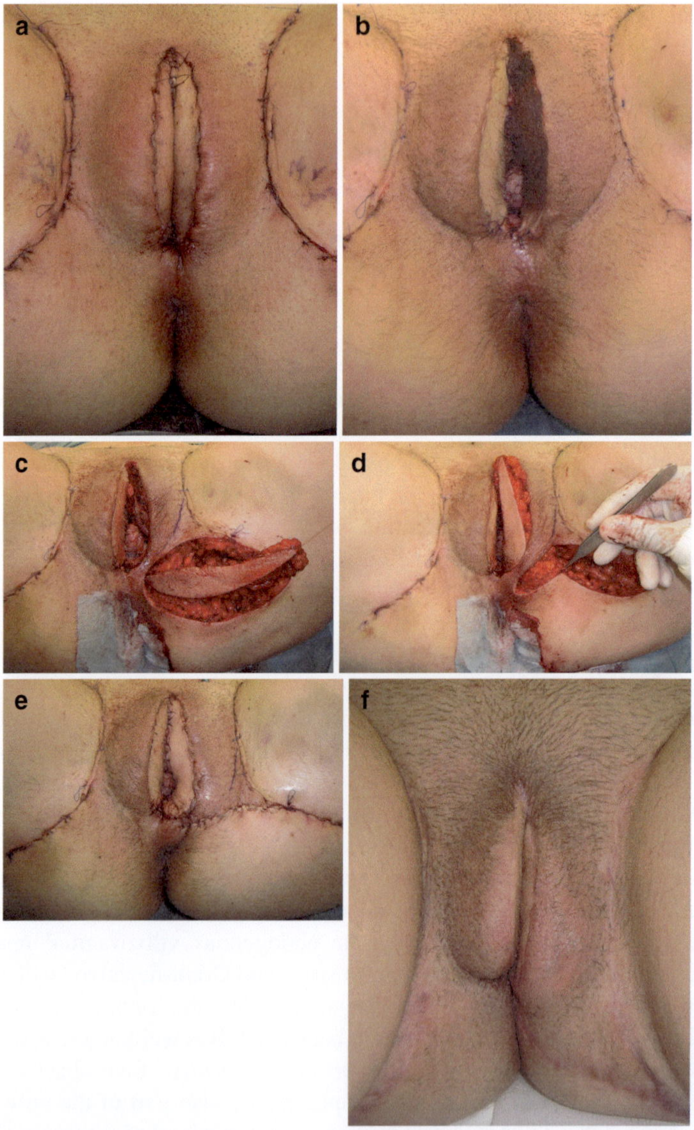

Fig. 3.19 Secondary vulvar reconstruction after left-sided aOAP-flap necrosis in a 30-year-old woman following lichen sclerosus et atrophicus. (**a**) (top left) Primary result after partial vulvectomy and immediate reconstruction with a both-sided aOAP flap; initial flap circulation was proper. (**b**) (top right) Follow-up after 7 days shows total flap necrosis of the left aOAP flap due to mechanical stress on the pedicle. (**c**) (middle left) Intraoperative view after removal of the necrotic left aOAP flap and harvest of a left-sided lipo-cutaneous flap supplied by the pudendal artery and vein raised from the femoro-gluteal region; note that the salvage flap borders the posterior aOAP-flap harvest side. (**d**) (middle right) Intraoperative view after transposition of the salvage flap into the left vestibule; harvest side is closed primarily. (**e**) (bottom left) Final result after completion of the flap procedure; note that the incisional concept of the salvage flap is coordinated to that of the former aOAP flap; so scarring is optimized even if it is extended. (**f**) (bottom right) Final result 9 months after surgery; note the still reasonable silhouette of the vulva even though scarring is extended and the posterior border of the salvage flap causes more bulk and likewise asymmetry at the posterior commissure

3.6.2.5 Vascular Insufficiency and Tissue Loss

Tissue loss following vascular insufficiency is one of the most feared complications in reconstructive flap surgery. It is known that initially after flap elevation the vascular capacity of the separated tissue block is decreased and likewise vulnerable. Original nutrient vessels except of the main perforator and auto-regulative nerves are excluded following flap harvest. This loss of inflow and sympathetic vasoconstrictor capacity lead to decreased perfusion pressure. Some systemic factors such as hypotension, smoking, or physical compression can additionally impair blood flow [17]. Regarding the aOAP flap, especially in obese patients, physical compression of the vascular pedicle over the inferior pubic bone might become relevant. The patient needs to relieve compression by spreading the legs for the first 3–5 days until flap autonomy is strengthened by inosculation from the flap bed. Fortunately, the aOAP flap is of a stable vasculature based on its reliable angiosome. It therefore does not tend to present vascular complications. As a fascio-cutaneous perforator flap it shows low metabolic requirements and should therefore be somewhat tolerant even for short periods of ischemia. A mobile and generous pedicle length ensuring tension-free transposition basically provides adequate flap survival.

In the rare case that relevant flap necrosis occurs operative revision is necessary. In case of total flap loss knowledge of salvage procedures is important (Fig. 3.19). Depending on the tissue conditions prevailed, a lipo-cutaneous flap of the femoro-gluteal region nourished by branches of the pudendal artery and vein is eligible to provide additional tissue for vulvar reconstruction. Due to topography the femoro-gluteal region is secondarily well combinable with the aOAP flap harvested out of the genitofemoral sulcus. Following that salvage procedure, increased scarring and a somewhat decreased reconstructive capacity will result.

3.6.2.6 Psychological Distress

FGM does influence body perception and sexuality of the affected individual. Even though body perception will be fit to the culturally imparted body image to a certain extent, most of the affected that I met do feel that there is something wrong with them. They almost always report on a dilemma between acceptance and rejection of the pathologic feedback they get from both their genital and their mind. “Acceptance” because they usually learned from their beloved parents and other people they trust what their own perception should regard as “normal.” “Rejection” because they usually feel that it is wrong to accept something, that they did not choose voluntarily, and that causes nothing but harm.

Currently, there are no standards established to address psychological distress in FGM/C victims, but many professionals do hardly work on it. However, I’m afraid it will be difficult if not nearly impossible to establish such standards, because FGM/C is closely linked to tradition, culture, and somewhat that might be described as “the unspoken.” “The unspoken” might be equated with ego, pride, honor, and other not measurable values that are worthy of protection for those being involved. Professionals dealing with FGM/C therefore should have an in-depth understanding of the relevant culture, values, and social interactions, and should provide strategies to maintain patient’s integration within their community. Besides the potential need for acute ease of psychological distress based on an impaired physical and/or emotional postoperative condition [18], long-lasting therapy might be necessary and potentially addresses a complex variety of tangible and supposed intangible factors of mind.

Sometimes problems following FGM/C are beyond anatomic needs and require psychological and social support. However, most of the FGM/C patients coming to my office already show a stable will to self-determination, and the fixed decision for reconstruction. That means that their decision has come a long way and that they clearly anticipate reconstruction with great hope to gain normality. They usually had had a lot of support from professionals and representatives and did a lot of mental work helping them to deal with their past and the major damages that were left by FGM/C.

Nevertheless, in case those patients feel compromised after reconstruction due to flashbacks linked to FGM/C, psychological support should be provided. Furthermore it might be advisable to provide support from a sexologist after reconstruction, because women may need to get guidance by learning how to use their newly received sensory capacity of their genital.

3.6.3 Secondary Complications

There are only few secondary complications that may occur several months after the initial operation. However, they may then surprise the patient, and also cause secondary interventions. These include negative scarring, and problems resulting from hair growth.

3.6.3.1 Scarring

Most contractures or indurated scars of the vulvar vestibule or the vaginal introitus are effectively treated with local massage, dilatation therapy, application of smoothing ointments, estrogen crème, and of course time. Surgical release might be necessary for refractory lesions or for contractures that are physically inaccessible for conservative treatment.

Besides adequate surgical planning and less traumatic dissections, application of local estrogen for a couple of weeks particularly supports vulvar wound healing and prevents for negative scarring. Clinically, local estrogen is proposed to induce collagen production and enhance epithelial cell turnover. Effective and prophylactic scar treatment, therefore, should clearly begin prior to scar development. I usually advice my patients after surgery to locally apply estrogen crème for up to 6 weeks in clitoral reconstruction and up to 12 weeks in vulvar reconstruction.

Scar-based stenosis of the vaginal introitus is usually not an issue unless the aOAP flaps are sutured together as a closed ring immediate in the midline anteriorly and posteriorly. So, even in extended cases, the risk of ring stenosis can be minimized by including an appropriate *bridge of vaginal skin* in between the aOAP flaps at the posterior commissure, or by generous *interlocking* of the flaps at the posterior commissure or rather at the perineum (Fig. 3.15).

In case, however, a ring stenosis occurs it can almost always be solved by conservative treatment using early dilatation, local massage, and estrogen crème over a period of 3 months. If a ring stenosis is resistant to those conservative treatments, scar revision is indicated. Scar excision and procedures like W-plasties, Z-plasties, or dancing-man plasties are very effective in the improvement of scar contractures of the vestibule and vaginal introitus.

3.6.3.2 Hair Growth of the Vestibule or Vaginal Introitus

To accomplish anatomic vulvar reconstruction it is important to address many details. Hair growth within the vaginal introitus or the inner vulva is not advantageous and may cause discomfort, and problems like skin irritations or dyspareunia. Unfortunately region of the genitofemoral sulcus is hairy in individual cases. However, hair growth associated with tissue transfer can be effectively removed primarily and secondarily by hair-targeted laser epilation such as high-powered diode lasers.

3.6.3.3 Folliculitis of the Vestibule or Vaginal Introitus

After reconstruction normal hygiene and regular wound cleaning usually prevent inflammation of hair follicles. In case that folliculitis occurs inflammation is typically limited and treatment does rarely require surgical intervention but local antiseptic and further cleaning treatments. If suture lines are involved, surgical revision might be indicated.

3.7 Personal Perspective and Epilog

First of all I would like to say thank you to all the courageous women (Fig. 3.20) able to insist on their immanent right of self-determination even though culture may not provide it for. Freedom and equality take a long way, but it will—and that's for sure—succeed one day in one way or another.

FGM/C is one out of several social errors existing in the world today. It reflects the objective to take sexual control of women, and to regulate their overall behavior. Even though reconstructive surgery cannot fix all problems associated with FGM/C, of course, but it can fix the anatomic damage left and thereby make an important contribution to end the impact of FGM/C in the individual. For the individual FGM/C is a life-changing procedure, but reconstructive surgery, and that is for sure, can anatomically bring back most of that what was taken.

After experiencing different methods for vulvar reconstruction while recognizing their intrinsic problems, I have come to the conclusion that women should profit from a more anatomic approach. That finding formed the basis for the development of my techniques for vulvar reconstruction represented by the OD flap, the NMCS procedure, and the aOAP flap (Fig. 3.21). Generally, reconstructive procedures should address both form and function to be differentiated from those techniques mostly effecting closure of a defect. In the end reconstructive procedures will almost always be rated to what extent they may or may not reach this goal [7, 19].

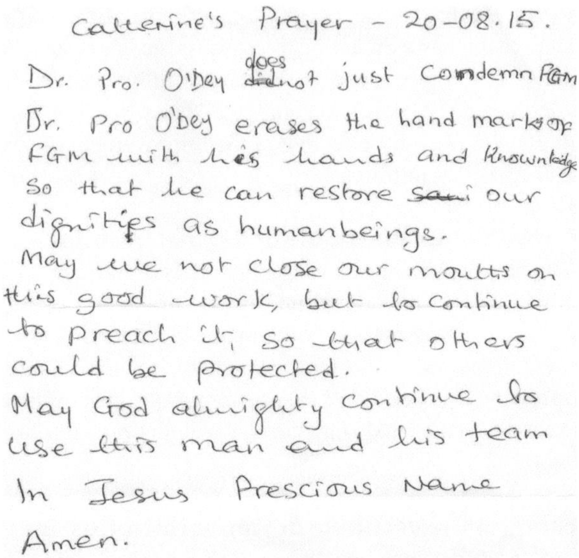

Catterine's Prayer - 20-08.15.

Dr. Pro. O'Dey does not just Condemn FGM
Dr. Pro O'Dey erases the hand marks of
FGM with his hands and knowledge
So that he can restore our
dignities as humanbeings.
May we not close our mouths on
this good work, but to continue
to preach it, so that others
could be protected.
May God almighty continue to
use this man and his team
In Jesus Prescious Name

Amen.

Fig. 3.20 "Catherine's prayer." Imagine the destructive impact of FGM/C on humans' psychological and physiological well-being and the creative significance of reconstructive surgery

Women suffering from FGM/C are severely burdened physically, socially, and emotionally. They suffer from relevant loss of genital perception, and overall loss of genital form and function. All these factors impair psychophysical balance, self-image, and body perception. FGM/C, therefore, is a complex issue and represents a major challenge to reconstructive surgeons and all the people engaged to abolish it. FGM/C patients frequently do not know how to describe their complaints, or feel themselves being hindered by tradition when they are directly asked to describe their genital problems clearly. On careful request, however, they usually start to describe the occurrence of pain typically in the context of menstruation and sexual intercourse. Furthermore they state the absence of sexual sensation. Sometimes it is necessary to anticipate their problems after clinical evaluation of their genital. Due to the fact that the strong will for bodily autonomy is progressive in women's minds, the number of women seeking for reconstruction is fortunately increasing. It is important, therefore, that reconstructive surgeons adapt or invent specialized techniques to always provide optimized procedures offering the highest benefits to affected women.

Other acquired deformities of the outer female genital deriving from different tissue or skin pathologies can show similar physical problems but have usually no cultural value to be respected. However, vulvar reconstruction following complete or partial vulvectomy as found in FGM/C patients or following other acquired deformities almost always represent a major challenge to reconstructive surgeons and all professionals involved.

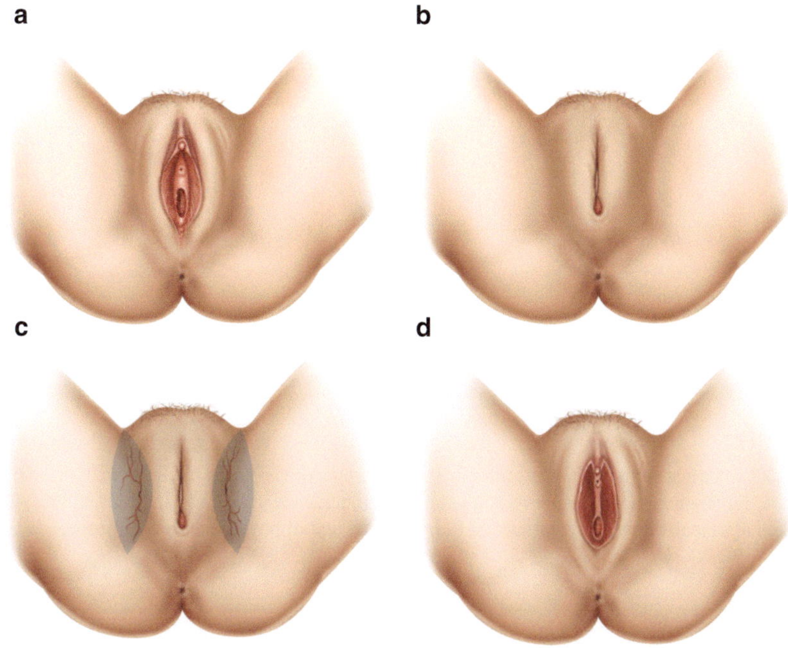

Fig. 3.21 Anatomic drawings of the outer female genital (*colorations of original drawings from the author*) demonstrating the dramatic change in anatomy before and after FGM/C III (infibulation) as well as the normalization following reconstruction. (**a**) (top left) Aspect of an anatomical normal vulva. (**b**) (top right) Aspect of a mutilated vulva following FGM/C type III (infibulation); note the disturbed anatomy and disabling closure of the vestibule. (**c**) (bottom left) Schematic planning of a both-sided aOAP flap; note the decentralized position of the perforator vessel and the anteriorly-posteriorly spanning extensions of the vessel. (**d**) (bottom right) Schematic result after complex vulvar reconstruction with the split-OD flap, NMCS procedure, and both-sided aOAP flap; note the reestablished shield-shaped form of the vulva due to the symmetric positioning of the aOAP flaps

All in all a comprehensive approach involving the people affected, human rights organizations against FGM/C and other nongovernmental organizations, governments itself, social workers, teachers, and health professionals like psychologists, gynecologists, urologists, pediatrics, and of course plastic surgeons is important to achieve the best for girls and women concerning the reconstruction of form and function of the outer female genital, reestablishment of physical and psychical autonomy, psychophysical stability, social integrity, and overall quality of life.

The key for all being involved to abandon FGM/C, however, is passion, persistence, and perseverance for a change (Fig. 3.22).

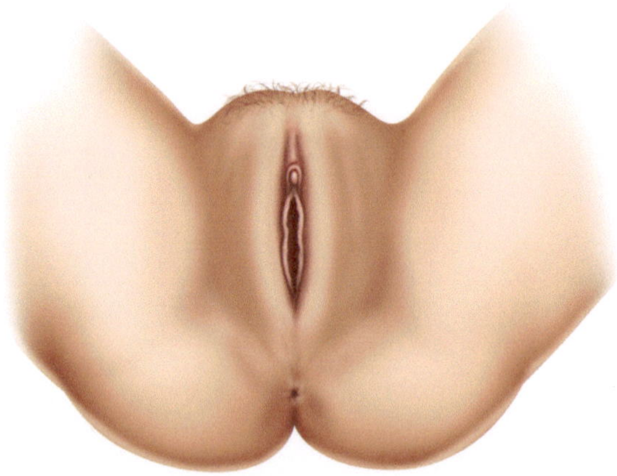

Fig. 3.22 "Vulvar reflection" (*coloration of an original drawing from the author*). Consider that the outer female genital is an important anatomic region in each individual, unique and versatile in detail, anatomically appealing, of special functionality, and of phylogenetic significance

Literature

1. O'Dey DM. Die rituelle Beschneidung der Klitorisregion: Anatomie und Wiederherstellung mittels Omega-Domed flap. Plast Chir. 2014;14(1):44–7.
2. O'Dey DM. Complex reconstruction of the vulva following female genital mutilation/cutting. Urologe. 2017;56(10):1298–301.
3. Madzou S, Ouédraogo CMR, Gillard P, Lefebvre-Lacoeuille C, Catala L, Sentilhes L, Descamps P. Chirurgie plastique reconstructice du clitoris après mutilations sexuelles. Ann Chir Plast Esthet. 2001;56:59–64.
4. Abdulcadir J, Tille JC, Petignat P. Management of painful clitoral neuroma after female genital mutilation/cutting. Reprod Health. 2017;14:22. https://doi.org/10.1186/s12978-017-0288-3.
5. Foldes P, Cuzin B, Andro A. Reconstructive surgery after female genital mutilation: a prospective cohort study. Lancet. 2012;380:134–41.
6. Foldes P. Reconstructive plastic surgery of the clitoris after sexual mutilation. Prog Urol. 2004;14:47–50.
7. O'Dey DM, Bozkurt A, Pallua N. The anterior Obturator Artery Perforator (aOAP) flap: surgical anatomy and application of a method for vulvar reconstruction. Gynecol Oncol. 2010;119:526–30. Epub 2010 Sep 24.
8. Chang TNJ, Lee CH, Lai CH, Wu CW, Chang CS, Cheng MH, Huang JJ. Profunda artery perforator for isolated vulvar defect reconstruction after oncological resection. J Surg Oncol. 2016;113:828–34.
9. Kim SW, Lee WM, Kim JT, Kim YH. Vulvar and vaginal reconstruction using the "angel wing" perforator-based island flap. Gynecol Oncol. 2015;137:380–5.
10. Lee PK, Choi MS, Ahn ST, Oh DY, Rhie JW, Han KT. Gluteal fold V-Y advancement flap for vulvar and vaginal reconstruction: a new flap. Plast Reconstr Surg. 2006;118:401–6.
11. Argenta PA, Lindsay R, Aldridge RB, Siddiqui N, Burton K, Telfer JRC. Vulvar reconstruction using the "lotus petal" fascio-cutaneous flap. Gynecol Oncol. 2013;131:726–9.
12. Huang JJ, Chang NJ, Chou HH, Wu CW, Abdelrahman M, Chen HY, Cheng MH. Pedicle perforator flaps for vulvar reconstruction—new generation of less invasive vulvar reconstruction with favorable results. Gynecol Oncol. 2015;137:66–72.

13. Windhofer C, Papp C, Staudach A, Michlits W. Local Fasciocutaneous infragluteal (FCI) flap for vulvar and vaginal reconstruction: a new technique in cancer surgery. Int J Gynecol Cancer. 2012;22:132–8.
14. Monstrey S, Blondeel P, Van Landhuyt K, Verpaele A, Tonnard P, Matton G. The versatility of the pudendal thigh fasciocutaneous flap used as an island flap. Plast Reconstr Surg. 2000;107:719–25.
15. Yii NW, Niranjan NS. Lotus petal flaps in vulvo-vaginal reconstruction. Br J Plast Surg. 1996;49:547–54.
16. Savada M, Kimata Y, Kasamatsu T, Yasumura T, Onda T, Yamada T, Tsunematsu R. Versatile lotus petal flap for vulvoperineal reconstruction after gynaecological ablative surgery. Gynecol Oncol. 2004;95:330–5.
17. Kerrigan CL, Wizman P, Hjortdal VE, Sampalis J. Global flap ischemia: a comparison of arterial versus venous etiology. Plast Reconstr Surg. 1994;93:1485–95; discussion 1496–7.
18. Abdulcadir J, Dimicheli FB, Willame A, Recordon N, Petignat P. Posttraumatic stress disorder relapse and clitoral reconstruction after female genital mutilation. Obstet Gynecol. 2017;129:371–6.
19. Höckel H, Dornhöfer N. Vulvovaginal reconstruction for neoplastic disease. Lancet Oncol. 2008;9:559–68.

MIX
Papier aus verantwortungsvollen Quellen
Paper from responsible sources
FSC® C105338

If you have any concerns about our products,
you can contact us on
ProductSafety@springernature.com

In case Publisher is established outside the EU,
the EU authorized representative is:
Springer Nature Customer Service Center GmbH
Europaplatz 3, 69115 Heidelberg, Germany

Printed by Libri Plureos GmbH
in Hamburg, Germany